Someone to Watch Over Me

by

Patricia Taylor

Someone to Watch Over Me

All Rights Reserved

Copyright © 2015 Patricia Taylor

Reproduction in any manner, in whole or in part,
in English or any other language, or otherwise,
without the written permission of the copyright holder is prohibited

For information address mickiedaltonbooks@lycos.com

First Printing 2017

ISBN: 978-0-6484766-8-9

Published by The Mickie Dalton Foundation
NSW
Australia

This book is dedicated to each of my precious and greatly adored grandchildren

Madeleine
Jack
Jazmine
Samuel
Chantelle
Hanna

because each of us has our own individual story and each story matters and is worth telling.

Acknowledgements

This book was born in my heart several years ago. My mother, Shirley would talk on and on during the many long telephone conversations I had with her, sharing her stories over and over again. I thought she would realise that she had already told me these stories, but I suspected that she drew comfort from the telling. Eventually I started recording excerpts on scraps of paper, backs of used envelopes, margins of letters and anything I could lay my hands on.

I decided one day to file these treasures away, dreaming that I may 'honour' my mother by writing her story. The day finally came and this book was written over a period of some twelve years. It has not been a solo effort, as several people have assisted me along the journey. Since its completion, it has remained for some years in a pretty, wall-papered box, awaiting the right time for tackling the challenge of turning it into a book.

Firstly I want to thank my husband Rob who has patiently endured all the lonely times as I've laboured on this project. Thanks dearest love for your faithful support whenever I have been in a spot on the computer and you have dropped everything to answer my pleas for help. Thanks also for taking on the huge challenge of helping with checking my spelling and re-arranging of sentences to make them clearer for the reader.

Thank you Michael Davies, my passionate and patient publisher. It has been a joy to work with you. Thank you Rose Good for introducing us.

Anne Van Loon, your loving encouragement and prayer has sustained me through some challenging times and strengthened me through the writing of this book. Thank you dear friend.

Dr. Robert Moles - former Adelaide University Law Professor and law expert - thank you Bob for answering my legal questions when I needed help for my book

A heartfelt thank you to each of my precious friends for your support and encouragement and patience as I have raved on about this book for twelve years. I treasure each one of you dearly.

Next I wish to convey my thanks to Dr David Buob, Principal Clinical Psychologist, who in his role as President, Glenside Hospital Historical Society, collated my grandmother Phyllis's medical records and prepared, very thoughtfully, a photo of my grandmother for the family. Thank you too, David, for your compassionate and generous offer of a phone call, and then an appointment, to discuss any of the contents in my grandmother's copious medical records. Your explanations and support were extremely helpful at a time when I needed to accept some difficult truths about my maternal grandmother.

Several years ago, whilst caravanning, I met the effervescent Ros Mills and her charming husband Tony. We enjoyed a candlelight dinner outside our caravan and swapped stories. I discovered that Ros was a proof-reader and the rest is history. I am so grateful to you, Ros for your expertise and support in editing this work. If I remember correctly, over a period of years, you have read this book four times. What a labour of love. Thanks from the bottom of my heart. You are a great friend and I love and appreciate you very much.

I was thrilled to discover you Sarah Brown as an ideal model for my front cover. Thank you so very much for your professionalism, patience, respectful attitude, enthusiasm and co-operation in regard to this project. I hope you like the end result as much as I do.

I also wish to acknowledge with a huge thank you my photographer, Gail Scholz, who also happens to be my daughter and therefore Shirley's granddaughter. Thank you Gail for your beautiful and professional work in "shooting" so many images so that we could get just the right one. I have always admired your skill in framing shots.

Next, I wish to acknowledge the heroine of this story, my mother, Shirley. When I first told her that I would like to write a book based on her story, she was very excited, even joyful. Her pleasure warmed my heart and I felt close to her as I sat at my computer, weeping over the details. As I write this I think of the complex and damaged person my mother became, because of the events that made up her individual life-story. Her enthusiasm for this book ebbed and flowed. I suspect that sharing her secrets in this way sometimes threatened her. I read excerpts to her and we talked about it on many occasions. She changed her mind several times and then eventually gave me her blessing. I explained to her that I wouldn't embarrass her by putting it into print whilst she was "with us." She was indeed a survivor and overcame the trauma of her early years in her own unique way.

Lastly I wish to acknowledge with deep love and gratitude my beloved Jesus Christ, who touched my spirit, broken and wounded from being raised by a broken and deeply wounded mother. His healing love brought me to a place of forgiveness for my mother and blessed us both with a truly loving and very close relationship during the last years of her life. I had the privilege and joy of leading her, after quite a battle, into acceptance of Him as her Lord and Saviour and as her beloved and very close friend. To hear her call out to Him often, professing her deep love and gratitude for loving and accepting her, and her joy that she would finally meet Him very soon, was always something that tugged at my heart and opened the flood gates of tears. What a merciful, gracious and compassionate God He is.

Shirley was many people in one skin, and this happened to her as a result of the abuses she suffered. Disassociation occurred, fracturing her personality, but enabling her to make the experience endurable. I will always love you my darling Mum. Your story lives on in my heart forever.

Author's Note

Some of the names in this biography have been changed.

Endorsement

In 2008, Ted Mullighan QC admitted he was taken aback by the sheer volume of people who were coming forward with life stories of sexual abuse to the inquiry he was conducting in South Australia, *"Children in State Care: Commission of Inquiry. Allegations of sexual* abuse *and death from criminal misconduct"* (2008). Shirley's story is one of these. Mr Mullighan recognised that the thousands of survivors he was listening to were 'the tip of a very large iceberg.' Shirley's story shows us the impact that abuse has on children and continues to have well into adulthood, and in fact Shirley carried it through into her old age. Shirley's story is an indictment on the justice and child protection system, which included the church, all of whom failed to protect her. It serves as a reminder of the precious children given to our community and highlights the right of each child to grow up in safety and flourish to maturity. For Christian teachers and workers it reminds us that we are always to reflect Jesus' love to children in our care, so they can become the people our God created them to be.

Patricia has documented her mother's true story with passion and clarity, making it an easy and engaging read. I highly recommend the book is read by everyone working with children, including health and care professionals, therapists, teachers, clergy, childcare workers and the judiciary. It is a story of human failure, yet through that failure shines the unfailing love of Jesus. That love continues to shine in Shirley's eldest daughter, Patricia, who has turned round a story that could so easily have become one of inter-generational trauma, into a story of compassionate love and support for her family and the many others who cross her life path. That's what Jesus can do!

Dr. Antonia van Loon BN, MN(Reasearch), PhD.

(Researcher working with survivors of child sexual abuse and author of *'Reclaiming Myself after Child Sexual Abuse,'*

'Facilitating Transition after Child Sexual Abuse' and 'Moving on after Child Sexual Abuse.'

Endorsement

What an honour to introduce you to the amazing author of this book!

Trish is effervescent, engaging, excitable, encouraging and most importantly, servant-hearted with a deep desire to empower women to reach their destiny! With an ability to draw others into connection, she skilfully encourages, equips and develops younger women to step up into their God-given abilities.

While travelling Australia in our caravan we landed at Emerald Beach NSW! During a communal breakfast at the caravan park, an older couple decided to join us. Rob and Trish quickly introduced themselves and before you knew it, we were deep in conversation about our encounters with God during this adventure round Oz. We quickly realised we shared the same love of the Father, compelled by conversations about our great big God!

Trish is a talented events co-ordinator with such a flare it's inspirational to all who look on at her accomplishments. Trish is pure joy. She is light and love to all who are blessed to spend time in her company. A calming balm to many souls.

Teeny Brumby
Alderman - Local Government
Tasmania

Endorsement

I first met Trish over the phone four years ago when she made contact with me after hearing my story on the radio.

Trish is an amazing woman of God who cares deeply about the wellbeing of others, and she works tirelessly in her efforts to enable the people she meets to live the best life they can. I am sure that Trish's passion has been greatly inspired by the uncovering of the story of her precious mother's tragic and devastating life as an abandoned child, living in an orphanage and on her own in the world.

Torn from her innocence at a young age Trish's mum Shirley endured a life of neglect, physical and emotional abuse, deprivation, starvation, imprisonment, child sexual abuse, slavery - involving sexual abuse, loneliness, and so much more.

I have had the privilege of staying with Trish and her husband Rob on two occasions and I have heard the heartbreaking story of her mother's horrendous and terrifying journey.

As Trish speaks of her mother I hear her voice soften and I see her eyes glisten as the grief of this story unfolds. This book has not only been well researched, but is beautifully written with such deep love and compassion for a mother who struggled her entire life just to survive, until she finally found a place of peace in the loving arms of Jesus.

As child abuse and neglect continue to affect so many in this world, I would recommend that all people (over the age of 15) read this compelling work.

Kerryn Redpath
Author: *'Out of the Darkness'* and *'Chasing After the Wind'*
Melbourne

Endorsement

The story of Shirley's life is a powerful testimony of the passage from Romans 8:37-39.

"No, in all these things we are more than conquerors through him who loved us. For I am convinced that neither death nor life, neither angels nor demons, neither the present nor the future, nor any powers, neither height nor depth, nor anything else in all creation, will be able to separate us from the love of God that is in Christ Jesus our Lord."

I remember sharing with Shirley and some of her family at her bed side at Eldercare Acacia Court, not long before she died. I encouraged them by saying... the best is still yet to come.... As Christian believers we have the wonderful promise from Scripture that if we believe in Jesus he will give us new resurrection bodies and we will be with him in heaven forever.

All the tears and crying and anguish and heartache and physical and emotional pain here on earth will pass away and Jesus will make everything new... The best is still yet to come!

Shirley was a wonderful lady who showed the love of Jesus to all she met while living as a resident at Acacia Court Hendon. It was a privilege to meet her and get to know her and it's a privilege to write this endorsement for the book "Someone to Watch Over Me."

Andrew Diprose (chaplain) – Eldercare – Acacia Court. 81 Tapley's Hill Road | Hendon | SA 5014

Endorsement

We were delighted to first meet Patricia Taylor and her husband Robert around 40 years ago when they came to the church in suburban **Adelaide**, South Australia, where I (Charles) was Associate Pastor.

Trish is a very talented woman who loves God and faithfully serves him in many different ways. Caring about others, and caring for others, is a large part of her life. And she has remained positive and committed to Christ throughout her life regardless of circumstances. One could describe her as living the Christian life on purpose. Christianity is not merely her profession, but is also what she intentionally lives out.

Trish has written her mother's story in a sensitive and caring manner which can encourage people who face huge obstacles in their lives.

Pastor Charles and Mavis Schwab
Geelong, Victoria, Australia

Endorsement

'Someone to Watch Over Me' is a moving personal account of the strength of the human spirit. This story of compassion and love, under tragic circumstances, needed to be told and more importantly, heard.

We all have a **responsibility** to care for all the vulnerable children in our society.

Rose Good
Author: 'Scheyville - The Last Camp'

Prologue

The icy wind had blown her hair all over the place and it looked the way she felt - a mess. Why had she done this? The question had gone over and over in her troubled mind. Why dig up the monsters from the dungeons of her past? She had tried to lock them behind heavy duty doors with bolts and padlocks for decades. Why had she stepped out into this ghastly weather and boarded a bus to hell? Was she finally mad - like her mother?

She shifted in her seat and pulled her padded jacket around her in order to zip it up and keep the chilly atmosphere out. The bus hurtled along the streets at an insane rate and she presumed the driver must be trying to make up lost time. He swung the bus around a corner and some of the passengers gasped as they tried to prevent themselves from being thrown into the aisle.

The elderly woman grabbed for the bar in front and at the back of the seat, flexing her thigh muscles to prevent a fall.

An agitated passenger called out, "Slow down for heaven's sake!" and others groaned in agreement. The driver threw caution to the wind and drove faster, obviously carrying a defiant disorder from his youth. Blood pressures rose and passengers stopped talking to each other, just hanging on, hoping to arrive alive.

She stared at her hands, not recognising them. They looked so old and wrinkled, with dark freckles here and there and purple veins standing up proudly. What had happened to those young and pretty hands of younger days?

Her hands looked like hands that had scrubbed floors, and nappies and dishes. Hands that had cooked and cleaned and washed thousands of plates and bowls without plastic gloves to protect from harsh chemicals and scourers. Weathered hands that could be read like a book. Hands that knew stormy days of drudgery and hardship. Hands that had not been pampered with manicures and delicately perfumed hand creams.

She wanted to stuff her hands in her pockets, but then realised she may make a spectacle of herself if she fell spread-eagled into the aisle. She hung on more firmly as that image caused her to wince.

"Who does he think 'e is? Jack Brabham? 'Es the worst driver I've had on this route." The woman next to her was sounding nervous but friendly. She glanced at her neighbour and saw that she was middle aged and wrapped in an oatmeal coloured three quarter jacket with a blue tartan scarf wrapped around her neck for warmth and woollen gloves that also grasped the bar in front.

"If we make it in one piece, I'm heading for Largs Bay. Where are you going?"

"I'm goin' on a bit further t' Taperoo. Wha' brings you to Largs?"

"I used to live there as a child. I'm just going past it to see if the place is still there."

"Is it a house on the esplanade?"

"Sort of. It's a very big house where lots of kids lived. An orphanage. I hated it. They were cruel to us kids."

Her neighbour didn't know what to say so she just said "Oh."

They travelled in silence for a long time. She stared out of the window, nervously looking for her first sight of the dreaded building. Suddenly she started to tremble. There it was. It was still there. The house of horrors. The place from hell. She grabbed tightly at the bar with both hands and stared at the place as the bus approached and sped quickly towards it.

"See that room at the top down the side there? That's the prison room. They put me in prison there and hardly gave me anything to eat or drink for days. A week. To punish me for running away. Witches they were. Wicked, wicked women in black. Bats. Evil and dark and cruel and they did everything in the name of the Father, the Son and the Holy Spirit they said."

"Were they all mean and cruel?" Her fellow passenger was Catholic and she was thinking of the lovely nuns she had known in her school days. Teachers who were mostly kind and thoughtful.

"There was one lovely nun - she was young and did what she could for us - as long as the others weren't around. They were bullies and she was scared of them. We all liked her and tried to do what we could for her. Some of them were worse than others. Much worse."

"Are ya' gettin' off the bus?" Her new friend was confused as to why there was no attempt from her troubled companion to move as they passed the building in question.

"No. I just wanted to see if it was still there. The memories have haunted me for years." Tears started to run down her face as the bats of dark memory rose from the basement of her mind.

She grabbed a handkerchief from her pocket and dabbed at the tears.

"I've never told anyone about those times. Not even my husband. I feel ashamed of what happened to me. Why would they be so horrible to innocent little kids when we didn't deserve it? What was wrong with us kids? Why didn't someone speak up for us and rescue us? Someone must have known................There was no-one to watch over us and care for us. We were absolutely alone.............. no one............."

Someone to Watch Over Me

Chapter One

Nineteen-Twenty Five

"Having children makes you no more a parent than having a piano makes you a pianist." Michael Levine

"I'm getting too old for this. Shut up you squawking little brat. Shut up I told you. You're driving me mad. What do you want from me? I've changed you, haven't I? I fed you before. Shut up. Shut up. Shut up. Stop screeching or I'll stop you for good."

Phyllis snatched up the tiny bundle from the drawer that was her bed. It was lined with old blanket pieces and torn up sheets and would suffice until the baby was big enough for a cot. The mother was angry and frustrated with her tiny offspring. Her patience had disappeared shortly after the tiny child had invaded her world with her demands. Phyllis felt there was no time for herself anymore, and she was untidy and grubby, just like her house. The frantic mother shook her screaming baby and shoved her face close to that of her unhappy child. The louder her mother screeched, the louder the distressed baby became.

Percy was at a loss. If he chided his wife, she would get worse, and maybe take it out on their little one. He should have left for work by now, and would need to step it out to get there on time.

His boss would accept no excuses for late arrival and with worsening news on the jobs front and predictions of higher levels of unemployment ahead, he had to be careful. Many were unemployed already and their families were going hungry. He couldn't let that happen to his little family. He'd better be going, but first he must try to calm his wife down.

"Here Phyllis, let me take her for awhile. You're frightening her with all that yelling. Go make yourself a nice cup of tea and cheer up love. Shirley is just needing a bit of peace and quiet, that's all."

"Calling me a bad mother, are you Percy? Don't you tell me what to do. She's the bad one, she is. Needs a good belting if you ask me. And I'm just the one to give it to her - for her own good. I'll show her. Just you get yourself off to work and I'll sort her out. She'll know who's boss when I'm finished with her."

Percy sighed and shrugged his shoulders. Work sounded a lot better than home these days, and he couldn't wait to escape. It was madness in this house and he didn't know what to do about it. He picked up his dripping-and-sauce sandwich which he'd made earlier, and kissed Phyllis on the cheek. He had made the mistake of forgetting before and there was hell to pay when he returned home. He wouldn't make that mistake again.

The icy wind was rattling the windows and hurling rain at them ferociously. He plucked his old grey coat and hat from the pegs near the front door and hurriedly put them on. He turned up the collar of his coat and wound his threadbare scarf around his neck, anticipating the onslaught when he opened the door. It was a cold August day and it would be freezing outside because of the icy wind and the relentless rain. He would walk briskly, and hopefully arrive on-time and not too saturated. He knew there would be a stack of work awaiting him and this would be a great distraction from his worries about things at home. There was a sudden even heavier downpour that beat noisily on their iron roof. He had no time to wait for it to ease off.

He glanced quickly at his tiny daughter, who was quiet now, hoping she would survive the day.

Chapter Two

"Life is like an ever-shifting kaleidoscope - a slight change, and all patterns alter." Susan Salzberg.

Percy had put in a good morning's work and his back was killing him. His boss had checked the chest of drawers he'd been working on and directed him to take a few minutes off to eat his lunch and get some fresh air. He was grateful to get outside because the air in the workshop was thick with fumes and he was coughing a lot.

He was a good French polisher and proud of his skill, putting his heart and soul into each piece of furniture. His work was demanding and it usually occupied his attention fully, allowing him to forget about his troubles for awhile. Today, however, the drawers from the chest reminded him of the drawer in which his little girl slept and his mind kept returning to his concerns about her and her safety.

His hunger pangs interrupted his thoughts and he sat down on the step and opened his lunch tin. It was bearable out here now that the rain had subsided and the wind had also died down. His sandwich was good. Anything would taste good to a man who was this hungry. Phyllis had not felt like getting tea last night and he had made fried bread. He'd soaked some stale bread in milk and then fried it in some left-over dripping they kept in an old jam tin behind the curtain under the kitchen sink. It was tasty with the meat juices from previous meals, but not enough of a meal for a hard-working man. He had fossicked around in the cupboard but couldn't find anything else to eat except some biscuits that his mother Florence had brought when visiting recently.

If only he had listened to his mother years ago when she'd warned him about Phyllis. Florence had observed she was not always truthful and suspected that she had lied about her age. Eventually he had found out his mother was correct and that his wife was actually six years older than she had told him. That made her thirty three, not twenty seven, when she married him. Even on their marriage certificate she had been dishonest. She had written twenty seven alongside his twenty two. Her eleven years seniority seemed to give her permission to be bossy and she certainly wore the pants in the marriage.

A baby had eluded them for ten years and life had been difficult with her, but, somehow he managed. Her hostility towards neighbours and friends, and his parents especially, had upset him, but as long as they kept to themselves, life was bearable. She drank too much and became loud and nasty, but other times she was pleasant enough.

Then there were the times when he was scared of her psychotic outbursts and the crazy things she said. Finally, when he thought it would never happen, she became pregnant. She also became crazier than ever. She was out of control, and her moods were all over the place. One minute she was laughing and then she was crying but mostly she was irritable. She was old at forty three to be having a first child, according to the mid-wife. Perhaps that explained her erratic behaviour.

His mother was conflicted over the news - so thrilled to be having a grandchild at last, but at the same time deeply concerned for the welfare of the child. He remembered another time when he had delivered news to her and had received a mixed reaction. It was eleven years ago. He had hurried home to their rented house in Stepney. He was still living at home with his parents, that is, when he wasn't away onboard the ship Limerick working as a steward. It was a warm and welcoming house, at the end of the street. The wide veranda was shaded by an old oak tree springing up in the front lawn. The tidy garden bore testament to a heart that cherished it and who toiled for hours, tending its patchwork of spectacular colour growing in the bordered garden beds. Rose bushes of differing heights and colour, daisy and lavender bushes, smiling sunflowers stood tall, and colourful petunias and geraniums of reds, pinks and pristine white splashed their colour around looking like an artist's creative palette. Butterflies fluttered in the sunshine, adding their touch of joy to a display pretty as a picture. There was an herbaceous border separating the plants from the gravel path and some elysium sat shyly at the base of the rose arch where floribunda roses in a vibrant pink threw caution to the wind in extravagant song. Even a casual glance informed the viewer that the inhabitants loved routine and order but did not sacrifice a variety of magnificent colour to accomplish control.

He raced excitedly through the back door of the house calling out to his mother to put the kettle on. Before the wire door had a chance to close, he had rushed into the kitchen and whisked her up in his arms and whirled her around the kitchen table.

"Good news, mother. I have great news. Where's father? He'll want to hear too."

Flo giggled with glee at her son's jubilation and couldn't wait to hear what he had to say. Her tight curls framed her plump and pleasant face, and her chubby cheeks shone bright pink without the need of rouge. Her prominent chin jutted out in a confident manner and she used it often, as she was well known in the neighbourhood for being a gossip.

"He's down the back collecting the eggs. It won't take him long. The hens have been a bit off their laying lately."

Flo started to fuss around with the kettle and cups and saucers, placing a cake on a plate and fumbling as she went, all of a dither about her only child's news. Arthur appeared eventually, in the doorway, obviously delighted to see his son home safe and sound. He was a good-looking man, but not really handsome. He had a strong, rugged look about his thick-set frame and you could see from the wrinkles around his eyes that he smiled and laughed often. His body had increased in size dramatically over the years and he blamed it on his wife's good cooking. His eyes twinkled and his moustache twitched as he greeted Percy.

"Sit down Arthur, our boy has news that he can't wait to tell us. Whatever is it Percival, don't make me wait a minute longer."

Florence was unable to keep her curiosity tamed any longer. Percival took a deep breath and fidgeted with his collar.

"Mother and father, I've met a lovely lady and I want to marry her." He blurted out the news and then sat down suddenly, hoping for a positive reaction.

"But you've been away on the ship working. However did you get time to meet someone and to spend enough time with her to get to know her enough to want to marry her?"

Florence's words were tumbling out all over the place, as she was both excited and apprehensive.

"It just happened mother, like in the movies. I was doing my work as a steward and looking handsome in my uniform (he gave her a cheeky wink) and there she was, a passenger, sophisticated and alone. Her name is Phyllis Carter and she is the most exciting woman I have ever met. She was travelling back from Melbourne where she'd lived for a few years with her mother and family. Her mother is a singer and has shared the stage with Dame Nellie Melba. Phyllis is very proud of her and indeed of all her family. She has a brother Charlie, and she wants me to meet him soon. He has his own business. They have always been very close. She thinks that he and I will get along very well."

"You want to marry this woman whom you've just met? Would it not be a good idea for your parents to meet her first?" said Arthur, a little concerned that his son was getting carried away and acting impulsively.

Someone to Watch Over Me

"I agree with your father Percival. We are pleased for you, but would like you to give this relationship some time. After all, you are only twenty two and have hardly had a steady girlfriend up until now."

"Phyllis is far too much of a woman of the world to be called a girlfriend, mother. She is marvellous. She has experienced so many things and she is very sure of herself. You will like her I am sure. She is very grown up and responsible."

His parents said no more on the subject except that they would look forward to meeting her soon. What a fool he had been to ignore their concerns when they did finally meet her. If only he had listened, he would not be in the situation that was giving him bone-jangling headaches now.

He had finished his sandwich and mug of tea and it was time to pull himself together and get back to his work. He would go and visit Charlie after work and have a brotherly chat with him. Charlie might have some helpful advice, having known Phyllis all of his forty years. Percy squared his shoulders, feeling much better now that he had a plan. He picked up his lunch tin and mug and headed back into the workshop and away from his problems for a few more hours.

Chapter Three

"My soul refuses to be satisfied so long as it is a helpless witness of a single wrong or a single misery. But it is not possible for me, a weak, frail, miserable being, to mend every wrong or to hold myself free of blame for all the wrong I see." Mahatma Gandhi

The two men sat in Charlie's front room. The house was in Cowandilla, about five hundred yards south of Henley Beach Road. It was a humble home, sadly devoid of furnishings. Charlie could barely afford to pay rent, so he settled for a roof over his head without concerning himself with too many creature comforts. The sitting room was just that. It was small, with an open fireplace and a couple of very old and sad-looking, threadbare armchairs. They came with the house and were a welcome comfort, replacing the packing cases which would have been the only other option.

Charlie was well known for the sparkle in his eye and his ready smile and cheeky greeting. He had an endearing knack of always expecting something good to turn up, no matter how bleak the circumstances. He dressed in the same jacket, trousers and baggy cap each day, changing his shirt for his only other one when it was grubby. He was a pleasant looking fellow, with a round face and glasses that perched on his chubby nose. Everyone liked Charlie. His personality was easy going and he was kind and generous when he saw someone in need. It was a mystery to those who knew him that he was still single and they

Someone to Watch Over Me

would jostle and tease him about this. Charlie was happy with the way things were, cherishing his freedom, and loving to go to the boxing for entertainment, and "the horses" when he had a bit of extra money in his pocket for a "flutter." He had seen enough of what a wife could do to a man in his sister's marriage to poor old Percy and he didn't want any of that for himself. He was a confirmed bachelor - in his late thirties - and would stay that way!

He had a green-grocery round, and he serviced his customers from early in the morning until well into the afternoon. He had to rise at four a.m. to harness old Blackie and they plodded off to market to pick up produce before the sun came up. It was as cold as charity in winter and they were both happy to return home at the end of a hard day's work. Times were tough for families and very often he would pull up at a place where food was needed, but money had run out. He was kind. Too kind for his own good according to Percy. Charlie would look at the hungry children, and let the mother take the food on credit. Sometimes he received payment later, and sometimes he did not.

He hardly made enough money to survive, but satisfied his hunger with left-over fruit and vegetables. He had become quite adept at making up a tantalising soup in a large, battered old saucepan that he'd had for years. He could not afford electricity, but always cooked over the open fireplace in the sitting room. He sometimes received payment for green groceries in armfuls of firewood, or eggs or sausages from the butcher, and this helped him get by. He had a pot of soup cooking now and the aroma made the men's stomachs cry out in hunger.

"Would you like to stay and have some of my hash soup with me Percy? You look like you could do with a good feed mate?"

"I am very tempted, Charlie. Phyl isn't too interested in preparing meals most nights. I usually have to throw something together at the last minute, when I get home. The cupboard is a bit empty at the moment, so goodness knows what we'll have tonight."

"Stay then. We can keep warm in there and have a bit of a yarn at the same time. I'll get some mugs and spoons."

"You've talked me into it. I can stay for a bit, but not too long. A bloke's life wouldn't be worth livin' if he got home too late. Not with her as cranky as she is these days."

Charlie gave his brother-in-law a knowing look and left to fetch the enamel mugs and a couple of spoons. Before long they were both warming their hands around the mugs and their stomachs with the delicious soup.

"Not bad. Whoever would have picked you as a good cook Charles? Sure beats what I'd get at home tonight."

They chatted for a while, Percy explaining to Charlie about his sister and her deterioration since the birth of tiny Shirley.

"I've noticed myself, mate. She's a cantankerous woman these days. Nearly bit my head off the other day over goodness knows what. I got out of there fast before she threw something at me.

"Probably a punch. Reckon she would make a good boxer. She's always looking for a fight these days. P'raps it's 'coz of the hard life she had as a child. She had it tough."

"She won't talk to me about it. Clams up. Must have been bad I reckon."

"It was. Our older brother Jack got out of the house and found work. The three of us, Phyllis, myself and little Adeline Rose lived alone after our dad died. He drank himself to an early grave. Mum drank too much too. She abandoned us and lived around the streets as a homeless person, picking up money for drink however she could."

He paused, thinking of things he didn't want to put into words. He stared at his mug, turning it around and around in his hands. Eventually he resumed his story.

Someone to Watch Over Me

"We tried to get by. It was hard. Now and again I had to pinch food for us so that we wouldn't starve. The neighbours helped out when they could, but eventually we found ourselves in court."

"They took you to court? Just kids? The stinkers! What did they charge you with?"

Percy was shocked.

"They charged us with being destitute children. Can you believe it? They threw us into the poor house. It was called The Magill Industrial School. Have you heard of it?"

Percy nodded, very slowly.

"Phyl was thirteen, I was ten and poor little Adeline Rose was only five. It was a very bad time for us. They dragged the girls from court. Screaming and kicking they were. Screaming my name. I'll never forget it. I have nightmares to this day about it.

"Charlie. Charlie. Help me Charlie."

"I was helpless. I tried to get away but they held onto me. I sobbed my heart out. We were close. Real close. Those "so and so's" wrestled us apart and we never saw each other again for years. It was a shocker. I asked to see them, when I got up the courage, but it fell on deaf ears. I asked if the girls were alright and no-one let me know. I was out of my mind with worry about what was happening to them. There were stories. Bad stories, and I just wanted to know how they were doing."

Percy could see that talking about it had affected Charlie badly and he was visibly upset. He didn't know what to say, so he said nothing.

"A few years later Mum pulled herself together and re-married. A German bloke. She got Adeline Rose and me released, but left Phyl there. Left her in prison actually. I think she was paid a bit for working in the laundry or something like that. Anyway, we went to live with Mum and our step-dad and their new baby. He was an ironworker and was away a lot in the country working. He sent a few bob back now and then, what he didn't drink - yeah, he drank too. I got whatever work I could, to keep us going. I went to visit Phyl now and again. She complained bitterly that she felt like she was in gaol and would never get out. When the place closed down she was sent to another to do laundry. She hated it. She wanted to know what wrong she had done to be treated like she was. She told me that horrible things happened to her there, and begged me to help her to escape. There was nothing I could do. I pleaded with Mum to get her out. She wasn't released though until she was eighteen. She was bitter and twisted over it. First chance she got she went and lived in Melbourne and looked for work there. Adeline Rose eventually joined her.

Charlie's voice trailed off into the distance at something Percy could not see.

"She must have been mad as hell at being left inside, after you two got out. That would stir up a saint. Poor Phyllis."

Percy was shaken by the story. He was also shocked that his wife had not shared it with him.

Both men sat staring into the fire for a long time. Percy sighed deeply. He didn't want to leave but knew he must. He thought of Shirley and felt guilty. He dragged himself away from the fire, put on his coat, hat and scarf and said his goodbyes to Charlie who was obviously saddened by their chat. Closing the door behind him, he trudged off with a heavy heart, heading for home and whatever awaited him.

Someone to Watch Over Me

Chapter Four

"God....rekindles burned out lives with fresh hope, restoring dignity and respect to their lives - a place in the sun." 1 Samuel 2: 7 - 8 The Message

Shirley was now three. Percy no longer lived with them. He was living with his parents, some miles away, in Payneham. He had lost his job, because there was not enough work coming in anymore. He picked up work wherever he could. Mostly he worked as a labourer.

He hated to think about the day he'd left Phyllis. It was the day he also left Shirley. The image was never far from his mind. Sweet Shirley with her big blue eyes brimming with tears, and then one huge tear overflowing and trickling down to her chin. She'd had her grubby little hand in his, hanging on until the last moment and then pulled it away, throwing both arms around his knees.

He'd looked down at her golden curls, sadly unwinding one and then watching it spring back into its curl. He had thought that the curl was just like her - always springing back, no matter what knocked her down and put her out of shape. He'd patted her on the shoulder. She had sobbed out words that he knew were pleadings for him to stay. Muffled words into his trousers. She lifted her troubled little face to look into his and tried again.

"Please don't go Daddy. Stay with me. Please."

He had slowly picked her up in his arms and held her for a long time. Phyllis had broken them up with nasty words. She spat them out at him and then dragged their child from him. Shirley struggled and squirmed to get free of her, kicking her little legs and crying out for her father.

"Just go, ya good for nothin'. Y're a boy, not a man. Get back to ya mummy and daddy and make 'em happy. No-one else would want ya - y're weak. Do ya hear me? Weak?"

Slowly Percy had picked up his kitbag with his few possessions, and walked away, the little one's screams piercing his head and his heart.

Yes, he was broken-hearted to leave the little one. They had always had a special connection, and she had cheered him up and made him laugh when things were grim all around him. She was a darling child and always rushed to him when he came home, lifting up her arms to be picked up, and then snuggling into his neck, forever.

But even Shirley could not make him stay any longer. Phyllis was more than unbearable. She taunted him day and night, reminding him of his short-comings and sneering at his attempts to show her love. Her mouth spilled poison and she beat him with her fists, or anything nearby when she became angry or frustrated. She was suspicious of everyone and constantly accused him of being unfaithful and of plotting to kill her. He'd had enough. He wanted out and he wanted his old life back.

He was worried sick that his disturbed wife would harm his child, but he quietly hoped and prayed that he could persuade his mother to eventually take in Shirley as well as himself. He felt certain that Phyllis's bizarre behaviour would finally cause her to lose custody of her daughter. He was worn out and on the verge of a complete breakdown. He comforted himself with the knowledge that Charlie would pop in each day and keep an eye on things. He was a good chap, Charlie.

Every two weeks or so, Percy would visit his child, and sometimes he would take her back to stay overnight with his parents. Once or twice they stayed with her great-grandmother Louisa Bradshaw, in Stepney. Florence and Louisa were close.

Someone to Watch Over Me

Louisa was a well-known and much loved character in the area. She had raised thirteen children herself, almost single-handedly, whilst running her own market gardening business and delivering many babies as the local midwife. Percy told himself that all the love these woman had to shower on Shirley would somehow help to make up for the horrible life she had with her mother.

Percy, like many of his contemporaries, could not afford a car. He caught tramcars, or he walked. Today however, his brother-in-law had loaned him Blackie and the cart.

"It will do the old boy good to take you there - better than standing around in the backyard all week-end."

Percy knew Charlie was thinking of his little niece and the fun that the trip would be for her, so he agreed. He'd picked up the horse and cart and had left it out the front of Phyllis's house, tied to a post.

There she is, in her usual place on the gas meter, waiting for me, he thought, with a tug at his heart. He reached over the fence and lifted her up into his arms. He could tell that she had been sobbing, hard. He held her close and felt her flinch in his arms.

"It hurts Daddy," was all she said. She kept catching her breath and clinging to him and he was at a loss as to what to do next.

As he turned around he saw Mrs. Sparks, the neighbour, come out of her front door and beckon him over. He complied and the friendly soul, with her navy pinny on over her blue dress with little pink flowers scattered all over it, ushered him through the front door.

"She won't hear us in here," she whispered, wiping her hands on her apron. "Hello little one" she said gently to Shirley. "Are you better now? You've had such a morning, haven't you? Mummy's been a bit upset, hasn't she?" Here let me take your little jacket off. I'm sorry, it hurts, doesn't it? What has she done to you this time? Eh? Let Daddy see. There we go."

Someone to Watch Over Me

Mrs. Sparks stepped back and let Percy take in the marks all over his little girl's arms. She lifted the little girl's dress and he saw, with deep shock, the same marks all over her thighs. Huge purple welts. She had been strapped with a belt, or something like that. Percy couldn't talk. He felt sick to his stomach. The child was three and a half. She had been whipped, mercilessly.

"Mummy hurted me," was all Shirley said.

Mrs. Sparks folded her arms on her ample bosom and looked firmly into Percy's face.

"You're the father. What do you intend to do about this? Either you do something or I'm going to report her. This poor child is going to be seriously injured one day, or, heaven forbid, killed. The woman is crazy. She flares out of control over nothing at all. She imagines most of it. And she's drinking too much. Some days little Shirley is so hungry she comes and knocks on my door and asks for food. She gobbles down what I give her fit to choke herself. It's not her fault. Her mother doesn't feed her properly. The other neighbours feed her too and we're all so worried about her. Can't you take her away to live with your parents before something terrible happens to her?"

Percy had no words. He nodded to the bearer of bad tidings and left her house. He carried Shirley over the dividing fence and to the front door of the place that he now called "the madhouse." He was angry. He dare not speak. He had to think. He had to get Shirley away without a scene. She had suffered too much today already. He'd known that things were bad for her, but had tried to put it out of his mind. Today, the truth of her mother's ill treatment was staring him in the face and he was shocked.

He knocked on the door. He felt like kicking it open and beating the life out of Phyllis, but what benefit would that be to his little daughter? He had to think. He had to grab her things and get out of there fast.

He heard his wife staggering to the door and knew she was drunk before he laid eyes on her.

Someone to Watch Over Me

"So, the hero Percy the prince is here to rescue his little princess from the nasty witch. 'Bout time. I was ready to send out a search par'y. She's been a pain in the backside all mornin' and I can't wait to see the back of 'er. Good riddance to both of yer. That's what I say. Get outa here and don't bring her back in a hurry. I can't stand the sight of her. Ugly little brat. That's what she is!"

She slurred her words and shoved a large brown paper bag into his hands. He guessed that it contained a change of clothes for Shirley. Her little dress was grubby, and she had wet her pants, but he dare not change her right away. They needed to escape quickly.

He noticed that Shirley had her fingers stuffed in her mouth, trying not to cry and she was trembling in his arms. He had not known until this moment that the little tyke was terrified of her own mother. He turned and walked away without speaking a word to his wife and jumped when he heard the door slam behind him. He quickly lifted his long legs over the low fence and then hurled Shirley and her meagre belongings onto the seat of the cart. He untied the horse and climbed up next to his little girl. He nestled her close to him, being gentle because of her injuries. He clicked his tongue and Blackie slowly took off. They headed into the sunshine and away from the storm.

Chapter Five

"Holding anger is a poison. It eats you from inside. We think that hating is a weapon that attacks the person who harmed us. But hatred is a curved blade. And the harm we do, we do to ourselves." Mitch Albom

"Rub a dub dub, three men in a tub" sang the tiny, curly-headed girl with the violet blue eyes. She was in the tub herself. It was a child's bathtub. Small and metal and oval shaped. Phyllis poured water in from the kettle that sat permanently on the old wood stove. She topped the bath up with cold water from the aluminium dipper that hung near the concrete trough in the lean-to laundry. When the mother thought the temperature was right for her little girl, she turned back to her stove, where she was cooking their tea.

It had been a very cold day, with gusts of wind that caused folk to scurry indoors and close their windows and curtains. Shirley loved the cozy feeling of being in a warm bath which her mother placed near the stove when the weather was particularly chilly.

This was one of those days when Phyllis's mood matched the weather. Her bad temper had been brewing all day, and Shirley had kept out of her way by playing outdoors, all wrapped up in her old coat and scarf. Finally her mother had called her indoors and she was loving the freedom of no clothes and the wonderful warmth of the water and the stove. Her spirits rose as she sang to herself, splashing and kicking and giggling with glee.

Someone to Watch Over Me

Shirley had been given a rare treat when she had recently visited her grandmother with her father. It was a cake of soap, all shiny and new and smelling of freshly picked flowers. Such luxuries were not experienced often in their poor household and Shirley made up a simple game that caused her to squeal and laugh out loud to herself.

The little girl squeezed the cake of soap until it slid, very slippery, through her pudgy little hands and back into the water with a 'plop' and a splash. She sang her little ditty over and over and continued to play with her cake of soap, making more and more noise. The neighbours loved to hear her sing because she had an exceptional voice and kept a tune very well. In fact, they were most surprised how many tunes she could remember with no difficulty at all. They ought not to have been surprised, of course, because music was in her genes on both her paternal and maternal sides.

Her father and grandfather played music together at district events, her grandfather being a well known violinist in Campbelltown. They also played regularly at their local Methodist church. Her beloved father played the organ, the bones, the flute and the bagpipes, honouring his Scottish heritage. Her grandmother on her mother's side, was a singer. She had performed on the stage and in 1909 had sung with Dame Nellie Melba during her sentimental Australian tour.

The food smelled good and Shirley knew it wouldn't be long before she would have to leave her tub and her singing and sit up at the table for tea. She felt very hungry, but she didn't want the fun to end either. Her mother was very angry and was drinking her beer and grumbling about the neighbours as she fried up sausages and eggs, which were swimming in deep, sizzling dripping in the blackened, old metal frypan. She'd had words with Mr. and Mrs. Sparks earlier in the day and had been annoyed with them ever since. The little girl wanted to forget about how angry her mother was, and sang at the top of her lungs and made her soap go higher and higher before it fell, splashing back into the now very soapy water.

Suddenly Phyllis turned sharply, the frypan in her hand, screaming at her child.

"Shut ya stupid cake 'ole. Ya noisy brat."

Her other hand held the egg slide which she waved to emphasise her words. Too late she saw that boiling fat had splashed out of the pan and into her small child's left eye. The poor little tyke screamed and yelled in agony as searing pain enveloped her. Shirley tore at her eye, trying frantically to get the hot fat out and to stop the pain. Savage pain. Blotting out everything else pain.

"Mummy! Mummy!" she screamed.

Phyllis knew that it was her fault, but in her drunken stupor and with a guilty conscience she turned on her chid.

"Ya stupid brat. I told ya to be quiet. But ya would'n listen. Ya wen' on and on enough ta upset a saint. Ya brought this on yarself. You're the one to blame 'ere, no-one else."

Phyllis would have gone on with her abuse had Shirley not passed out. As drunk as she was, she pulled her child clumsily from the water, or she would have drowned. Phyllis wrapped her in a grubby towel and placed her on her bed. She stood staring at her, not knowing what to do, frozen to the spot. The door suddenly burst open.

Phyllis turned to see Mrs. Sparks standing there holding the hand of her little eight year old son Tom. They both looked shocked as they looked at the still little form lying wrapped in the towel, on the bed.

"What have you done to her?" screamed Tom, looking like he was going to kick the drunken mother in the shins.

"Easy Tom. Let Mrs. Gilfillan tell us what has happened." Mrs. Sparks eased herself over to the small child, trying to position herself between her and her abusive mother.

Someone to Watch Over Me

Shirley woke up. The shocking pain caused her to scream again. She frantically rubbed at her eye but it only made it hurt all the more. Her mother screeched at her to stop, grabbing her hand away from her injured eye. Mrs. Sparks tried to calm Phyllis, but eventually gave up and put her arms around the distraught woman, effectively restraining her, all the time steering her to the kitchen for a "nice cup of tea."

The kettle was filled and moved back onto the wood stove, and Phyllis was seated at the kitchen table, before Mrs. Sparks quickly returned to the distressed child. She needed to work out what had happened and knew that it was no use asking the child's drunken mother.

Mrs. Sparks and Tom had heard the singing next door and then the screaming and yelling. She saw the upturned frypan on the kitchen floor, the bathtub near the stove, and did not need to be Sherlock Holmes to work out what had happened. She gently cradled the injured little girl in her arms as she instructed her son to run for his life to Dr. Johnson's place and then on to Shirley's Uncle Charlie's house. She knew that it was quite a distance, but Tom was a fit boy and he loved this poor child like a sister.

Mrs. Sparks heard the kettle whistling and ordered Phyllis to make a cup of tea. She hoped that this would give the woman something to do and distract her further from her unhappy little girl. The mother's yelling only added to the child's distress, frightening her even more.

Dr. Johnson came straight away on his bike, with his bag of lotions and potions in hand. He quickly explained that Tom had run onto Charlie's house and that they would hopefully arrive in the next few minutes, should Charlie be at home. He squatted down by the tiny child who was sobbing as her kindly neighbour held her tightly in her arms, trapping both her hands from rubbing at her poor eye. The doctor looked very concerned as he pried her eye open and tried to see what damage may have been done. Phyllis stood nearby, with a mug of tea in her hands, watching silently now. Mrs. Sparks explained what had happened and the old family doctor frowned at Phyllis and glared without words, his black look speaking for him.

The mother had finally grasped the gravity of the situation and that the injury to her child's eye may be permanent. The events of the last hour had sobered her considerably and she stood staring at her tiny offspring with deep furrows across her forehead.

The kitchen door flew open again, and this time a very anxious Charlie came running into the room, heading straight for Shirley's bedroom, off the kitchen. He fell to his knees alongside the bed where Shirley was lying quietly now. Dr. Johnson had given her something to ease the pain and to help her to sleep. Charlie searched the doctor's face for an answer to his unspoken questions. Young Tom was struggling to catch his breath and came in just behind Charlie. He eased forward, wanting to know how bad the injury was, and if his little play-mate's eyesight in her left eye might be lost.

The doctor shook his head from side to side. He explained that the boiling fat had more than likely damaged her left eye permanently and there was nothing he could do to prevent this outcome. Everyone in the room stood silently, deeply saddened by this news and hoping and praying that this would not be so for this lovely, innocent little child. There was no sympathy in the room for the bad tempered, drunken mother who had caused it.

Sadly, the doctor was correct and Shirley was blinded permanently in her injured eye. The colour faded as well, to a very pale and milky blue. Whenever she asked Charlie about her "bad" eye he would only ever answer gravely:

"A little bit of fat got in it Shirley. A little bit of fat."

No matter how she pleaded, he would say nothing further.

Chapter Six

"Temper is a weapon that we hold by the blade."

'Knock, knock.'

Shirley was sure she had heard someone at the door. She told her mother, but was ignored.

'Knock, knock, knock.'

Shirley pulled herself up carefully and went over to her mother.

"Someone's at the door," she whispered, and then breathed in quickly, like a short gasp.

Her mother had belted her very badly this time and she had been crying a lot. She was scared that Phyllis would start up again. When her mother did not respond and the knocking kept up, she walked down the long, dark, narrow passage-way to the front door. It had pretty, coloured glass around the door, and let in light during the day. It was very dark outside now, so Shirley stretched up as far as she could, and managed to switch on the outside light.

She had no idea who the visitor might be because anyone they knew usually just walked around to the back door which opened to a porch and then into the kitchen. Everyone just called out and walked in. She cheered herself up with the thought, even so, that it might be one of their neighbours calling to see if she was alright. They were her friends, even though they were grown ups and she was just "a little flea" as they affectionately called her.

Someone to Watch Over Me

Two ladies were standing there on the tiny veranda. They were strangers to her. They were dressed in uniform.

"What is your name little girl?" one of the ladies asked her, bluntly.

"Shirley," she replied. "What's yours?"

The woman ignored the question and asked another.

"Is your mother at home Shirley?"

"Yeah she is," said Shirley.

The other lady was taller, but softer, and she bobbed down on her haunches and gently asked Shirley to get her mother for them. Shirley didn't move. She looked down at her feet.

"What's wrong little one? Don't you want to get your mummy? Are you sure she is at home?"

"Yeah. She's cross though."

"So we heard," said the first woman sharply.

"Do you think you could take us to your mother Shirley? We want to talk with her."

Shirley didn't answer. The little girl had learned not to tell anyone about her mother.

The tall, soft lady, still squatting at Shirley's level, put her hand gently on the little girl's arm. Shirley flinched. The policewoman quickly withdrew her hand, realising that the child was hurt.

"Do you think you could point and tell us where your mummy is Shirley? We may be able to help her."

Shirley nodded and pointed to where a light was on at the end of the long passage-way.

"How old are you little one?"

"I'm not little anymore. I'm big enough to milk Bessie now. I'm four." She spoke the words with such pride that the two policewomen were touched.

They did not miss the catch in her breath when she spoke. It was easy to notice that their little guide had been crying very hard.

"Is Bessie a cow?" asked the shorter woman, not to be outdone by her companion, in winning over the child.

"Yeah. Daddy bought her for us so that I would get plenty of milk for my teeth and bones."

The child had an opportunity for pride with these two adults, at last.

Finally the three arrived at the kitchen, and the illumination from the single fly-speckled globe hanging from the centre of the room revealed that Shirley was not only upset, but filthy. Her hair was matted and there were large, purple welts on her tiny arms.

"Wha' you two coppers gawking a'?" came the voice from the mess in the chair.

"Are you Phyllis Gilfillan?" said the policewoman.

"Who wants t' know an' wha' are you two coppers doin' in me 'ouse?" asked Phyllis.

"We've received complaints again that this little girl is being mistreated and we have come to investigate," was the solemn answer. The woman braced herself for the onslaught. She was not disappointed. Phyllis gave her a mouthful of abuse and would have hit her if the police-woman hadn't cautioned her severely.

"We need Shirley to take off her dress please Phyllis. Could you do that for us please little one?"

Shirley looked frightened and looked at her mother.

"It's alright darling. We just want to have a look at your back."

She looked at Phyllis who kept quiet now. Shirley took off her dress very slowly. Her hands were shaking and it was clear that it hurt her to do so. Both the women gasped as they saw her little body covered in huge welts. Welts that stood proud, purple and angry. Here and there the skin had been broken by the vicious belting that had been inflicted on her tender skin. Her torso had taken lashings, front and back, and there were marks on her thighs as well as her arms and hands. The women looked at each other, ashen-faced, and nodded in agreement.

Someone to Watch Over Me

"Phyllis, you are an unfit mother and this child is being severely mistreated. You don't deserve to have a child. You are drunk and dirty and a disgrace. We are taking Shirley away from you, giving her a good feed, and then a doctor will examine her and attend to the damage that you've done. We will have to see about her future when you are in a better state to give us details."

Shirley started to protest. She wanted her Uncle Charlie. She wanted her grandma, her daddy. She didn't want to be taken away by strangers. She didn't know where they were taking her.

"Help me mummy, help me," she pleaded.

"I'm sorry I let them in. Don't let them take me away."

Her mother remained in her chair and shrugged her shoulders as she picked up her beer.

"Ge' outa me 'ouse before I throw yas out!"

"We need to take your child with us for her protection."

"Ova ma dead body!" yelled Phyllis.

"You are the worst mother I've ever seen. This poor child has been beaten cruelly. She is defenceless and helpless and only four years old. You are disgraceful. She looks like she could do with a good feed too. Yet you seem to have enough money to supply yourself with beer, and I'm guessing that's where most of the money is....."

The policewoman did not finish as Phyllis jumped out of her chair and threw herself at her, with the beer bottle threateningly in her hand, screaming obscenities. The other police officer rushed forward and the two women wrestled the bottle away from her and held her down in her chair, kicking and screaming abuse. They all momentarily forgot the traumatised little girl who stood there with eyes wide open, staring at the terrible scene. She felt responsible, having let the two women in. Her mother was always saying "I'll kill ya if ya don't do what I say." This time it would happen for sure. She ran screaming from the kitchen and into her bedroom and threw herself under her bed. With her eyes screwed tight and her hands over her ears, she tried to block out of her world the feeling that something very final was taking place in the kitchen. Eventually someone came in to her room. She gently persuaded Shirley to come out from under the bed as she placed a few of her things into a large brown paper bag she had found in the kitchen. Shirley was reassured that her uncle, father and grandmother would be contacted on the following day and they would work out what to do with her. This encouraged the frightened little girl and she picked up her shoes and put them on.

    Saying goodbye to her mother was deeply distressing for the tyke. Shirley was worried for her, and yet scared of her as well. She gingerly went up to peck her on the cheek and was amazed when Phyllis grabbed her and hugged her to her huge bosom, sobbing and crying out her name. Shirley was too shocked to cry and walked slowly away with her hand in the hand of the authority figure who led her into the dark and the unknown.

Chapter Seven

*"It takes a lot of loving to make a house a home.
Not paint and decoration, not mortar, bricks or stone.
It takes a lot of laughter, in sunshine times and shade,
Of treasuring the things within, no matter the price you paid.
It takes a little miracle that only love can do -
To take a humble house and make a cherished home for you."*

Patricia Taylor

Shirley's great grandmother was a saint, according to the locals. She had been a bit like "the old woman who'd lived in a shoe and had so many children she didn't know what to do," or so Florence used to say. She had been a hard worker, raising thirteen surviving children and running her own market garden at Campbelltown. She was a popular and familiar sight for the locals, sitting outside her shed, shelling the almonds that she had just knocked on to an old sheet with a broom. She had two concrete troughs in the open and she would wash the vegetables, ready for carting and sale. Sometimes the weather was overbearing because of the heat and at other times it was bitterly cold. That was part of living in Adelaide where the seasons would bring boiling hot summers and freezing cold winters. Louisa persevered, shrugging off discomfort and completing the task. When the almonds were shelled, or the fruit and vegetables prepared, she would beckon her faithful old horse Fred, harness him, attach the cart, fill it with the fruits of her labour and then they would trudge to the East-End Market in the city of Adelaide. Here she would set about selling her produce.

This romantic market garden had been the setting for the first time meeting of Florence and Arthur, the love of her life. He had come to work for Louisa and Thomas Bratchell (later changed to Bradshaw). He had found favour with Louisa because he too was a hard worker and not a shirker like her husband Thomas. Sadly, her husband had never been interested in work, but soon learned that Louisa could not stand a job undone and would pick up the slack for him. In fairness to Thomas, he was often not well with bronchitis and asthma and would sometimes be seen hanging over the fence, struggling to get his breath. He was missing for long periods of time as he also worked now and again as a bullocky, to bring in extra money and to escape all the kids and duties at home, according to the neighbours.

Louisa was a well-loved person in that close-knit neighbourhood. She was known not only for her amazing work ethic, but also for her kindness and generosity, even when she could ill afford it. In spite of her huge work load, she was a mid-wife and delivered many of the local babies. She was a popular mid-wife because she empathised with the mother in her pain and anxiety, having given birth to so many babies herself. Shirley's great grandmother was feisty when it came to her family and their welfare. At one stage there was an altercation with the local baker over a loaf of bread. Louisa wanted it on credit, offering to pay when she had cash from the sale of her produce in the market. He would not agree and Louisa made her own bread until he relented. He eventually gave in because Louisa bought a lot of bread for her large and hungry family.

When Thomas died, in spite of all her exhausting work, Louisa was left a very poor widow. Thomas, true to form, had not left a will and this caused complications for Louisa. She had many children to raise and feed, and a market garden to run.

However, this did not stop her from giving away more fruit and vegetables than she could afford. Reluctantly she had to face the reality of their hardship. Having to accept the pension to survive distressed her immensely as she thought it was a disgrace to do so. Louisa thought that everyone should be able to support themselves and felt like a failure for needing to rely on a "hand-out."

Her mud house with thatched roof was her pride and joy, in spite of the lack of furniture. She kept it as neat as she could, delegating chores to her offspring. It perched prettily in the well-tended cottage garden, rows of oleander shrubs in the background and various fruit trees creating shade and contrast. There were little walks everywhere, taking visitors on meandering treasure hunts, with many varieties of vegetation to discover and enjoy. There were roses of every hue, splashing colour everywhere, both on bushes and poles and climbing up walls and cascading from the thatched roof. Iceland poppies peeped out cheekily from behind lavender and daisy bushes and impressive hollyhocks were standing tall, yet leaning at precarious angles throughout the garden, displaying many different shades of pink and red. Magnificent delphiniums, bathed in purply blue added their statement when it was their time to perform, and brilliant golden sunflowers sang their song without self-consciousness, each year. A favourite with visitors were the bird of paradise bushes with their colourful floral "birds" whenever they made their enchanting display. In shaded spots, under fruit trees, appeared colourful hydrangeas with heads as big as cauliflowers, and nearby were glorious yet humble geraniums and pelargoniums, competing with each other to produce the brightest bloom. Louisa loved to take cuttings from these species to give to neighbours and friends. It gave her great pleasure to know that her plants would go on and on giving joy all around the neighbourhood.

Someone to Watch Over Me

Beautiful Nance, as she was known to the locals, was indeed pretty and sweet-natured. Her real name was Sarah Ann, but even her tombstone read Nance Bratchell. She was the most delicate of the daughters of Louisa and Thomas, suffering from a heart condition and asthma. It was her duty to tend the garden and each day she would be seen from dawn until dusk, working diligently amongst her beloved plants. Her gentle nature caused her to often give a bunch of flowers where there was a need and this endeared her to the locals. Young Nance loved each plant and was especially fond of the Iceland poppies. They were just about to bloom when Nance sadly passed away at fifty-eight years of age from Acute Peritonitis following Appendicitis. Many times the old adage "only the good die young" was passed from neighbour to neighbour as they grieved her passing. The picture of such beauty tending a magnificent garden with gentle grace and kind greetings to those who passed, was a snapshot left in their hearts for the rest of their lives.

Many edible fruits were produced in this garden, including cherries, persimmons, grapes and mulberries, and of course the already mentioned almonds.

Flo and Arthur's romance developed in this idyllic setting and they married and had one child, Percival. Their only grandchild was Shirley. Sadly, Arthur did not get to meet her because he passed away four years before she was born. Flo idealised Arthur and never got over losing him. She lived for several years with her mother Louisa, who remained a hard worker even though aged and frail and in need of a walking stick, and later a wheel chair.

Louisa died in 1929, the year that Shirley was taken from her mother by the two women police officers. Flo was very distressed about the loss of her beloved mother and was heart-broken and inconsolable for a very long time. This interesting patch of turf has housed some other fascinating people. It was sold when Louisa died and changed hands a couple of times until Tony Sabino and his parents arrived from Northern Italy and purchased it. They set to work. Hard work. They were market gardeners too, and they carried on with the same spirit of grit and determination that Louisa had. She would have been impressed. By then Louisa's old mud house had traded its thatched roof for a corrugated iron one and an outside washroom had been built on as an added luxury.

Indomitable Louisa had created a beautiful home in a very small, one roomed cottage. A home where the walls hid many memories of love and laughter, fights ad tears, hopes and dreams, shared chores and family togetherness.

As fate would have it, young Shirley did not find herself taken into the sanctuary that Louisa's family would have provided. Instead of paths bordered with colourful annuals, hers were barren and bleak and storms continued to threaten.

Footnote

The Sabino family lived happily in Louisa's old house until a flood came through the area and damaged it beyond repair. It needed to be demolished and Tony Sabino sentimentally sketched his home before it was destroyed. To this day the neighbours look forward to Louisa's mulberry bush bearing fruit for them to collect each year.

Someone to Watch Over Me

Chapter Eight

"Too often we underestimate the power of a touch, a smile, a kind word, a listening ear, an honest compliment or the smallest act of caring, all of which have the potential to turn a life around." Leo Buscaglia

Shirley's mother Phyllis was now living in an institution, unable to care for herself, and considered 'hostile and dangerous'. She was mentally ill, her own tragic life experiences having sent her 'over the edge.' She was to spend the rest of her life as a patient at the Parkside Mental Hospital (later called Glenside Mental Hospital), apart from the last two years where she saw her days out at Northfield Mental Hospital. The tragedy for her was worsened by the fact that she'd spent most of her life institutionalised, both as a child from thirteen until eighteen, and then as an adult from when Shirley was four until she passed away at seventy nine years of age on the eleventh of October, 1962. Her heavy drinking may well have been a symptom of her hardships and she quite obviously inherited a propensity to addiction from both parents. This drinking problem probably contributed to her mental illnesses and her psychotic behaviour.

Her life was therefore terribly sad and her existence a miserable one in 'Parkside' where conditions at the time were shocking. The living quarters consisted of one-person "cells" where there were no pictures on walls, curtains at windows, or lockers, a table or even a chair. Escalating numbers meant two persons shared the one-person cell or the alternative was a frightening, overcrowded ward. Clothes belonged to no-one, but everyone. Consequently all clothes were shared and this resulted in ill-fitting, unsuitable garments for the patients. The indignities of their environment were depressing and conducive to low morale. The place was shamefully understaffed, and the recreation rooms were far too small and ill-equipped for the number of patients. In fact, over-crowding was at a dangerous level, and recreational activities at a bare minimum. "Doom and Gloom" would have been a good nickname for the place.

Phyllis had thyroid disease as well and this was not understood or diagnosed and therefore not treated for many years. Dr. A.S. Czechowicz, who was superintendent of Hillcrest Hospital (formerly called Northfield Mental Hospital) informed family members after Phyllis's passing that it was a tragedy for Phyllis that thyroid disease was not understood back in those days. Phyllis may have been able to be treated and then live in the community with her child. Instead, she suffered from unpleasant symptoms including severe hair loss, resulting in her need to wear a "beanie" to keep her head warm, obesity, depression, and constipation. Percy waited many years before divorcing her. One can only imagine the guilt he battled at taking the final step of separating from her in the divorce court.

Grandmother Louisa was now frail, and she lived with Flo as well. The younger woman was very opinionated and was often annoyed with Percy for abandoning his only child. But her annoyance eventually abated. He was, after all, her only child, and the sunshine in her day, with her husband Arthur having passed on. Percy was now the object of her affection, and his small child was doted on by her. She fussed over her mother as well and the two women competed in pampering Shirley. They both liked to dress her up like a little doll and they had a friend who painted a portrait of her in her best shell-pink dress with her hair in curls. Prior to the sitting for the portrait, Shirley had endured a practice common in those times of having her hair twirled in rag strips to produce long springy ringlets, emulating her idol, Shirley Temple.

Her favourite times of all were when her daddy would play an instrument and she would sing. Visitors were treated to these impromptu musical moments and would often sit speechless and spell-bound. Shirley knew that her daddy was very proud of her and it made her extremely happy when he would kiss her on the cheek and say so.

Florence Gilfillan liked to think that she was a real lady. Whilst her mother had worked hard at making a living, Flo worked hard at making an impression. She lived in a 'nice' house, even though it was rented, in a 'nice' area, and her husband had belonged to 'The Lodge' and the church and had been very much respected in the St. Peters district. His talent as a musician had been greatly appreciated. His funeral had been huge, with many notices about his death in the newspapers. In fact, notices in the newspaper were very important to Flo and she continued to place memorial notices for many years following his death. Her son's name was also included with hers and Shirley's except for one year when she was very angry with Percival and he was excluded. Florence was a great one at keeping up appearances and was very much like 'Hyacinth Bucket', who pronounced her surname 'Bouquet' from the popular TV series 'Keeping up Appearances'.

At first she loved having little Shirley around for company, especially because Percy moved in as well. However, she was a terrible gossip and spoke too openly about the circumstances that brought Shirley to live with her. Flo loved the attention, fuss and praise that the story brought from friends and neighbours, until she overheard what was being said behind her back. When she thought things through, she realised that she would have made the same hurtful comments, had the story been someone else's and not that of her own little grandchild.

This took the shine off having Shirley living with her. Also, the little girl had emotional problems and often burst into tears for no apparent reason. She saw the whispers behind raised hands in church and in the street. Flo noticed sympathy replace admiration. It was hard to keep up appearances and play the lady of St. Peters anymore. It was hard work looking after a four year old, as well. She was ashamed of her son's crazy wife, and of his abandoning his family. She felt that she was being used by him and that she had lost her freedom. Resentment set in and she and Percy argued often.

With Louisa's death, part of Florrie died with her. It was not until she lost her mother that she realised how very much she had depended on her all of her life. Louisa's grit, indomitable spirit and sheer goodness of heart sweetened her life and made it bearable. Suddenly the sweetness was gone. Flo was lost, alone and without comfort. For a while she clung to little Shirley and tried to throw herself into looking after her and Percy. Her son was out each day working from early until late, as a labourer. When he came in at night he was exhausted and no company for her. It became all too hard for Flo and she wanted a life of her own.

Phyllis was allowed out of the mental home a couple of times on trial and Shirley went to visit with her. Charlie moved into Phyllis's old house on Henley Beach Road, to keep an eye on things, and social workers visited to check on Phyllis as well. She was subdued and managed to keep herself reasonably clean and sober. Shirley loved being with her mother on these visits and remembered for the rest of her life the long walks, on little legs, to visit her uncle's grave in the West Terrace Cemetery on the western side. Jack was the adored older brother of Phyllis and Charlie. They were very proud of his being one of the brave Australian Light Horsemen. He was with the Twenty-fifth Regiment and embarked in December, 1916. He had somehow miraculously survived the First World War, and returned home to Adelaide to live. He died in April, 1929, the same year Phyllis lost control of her life, and lost Shirley as well. His death had been the last straw for her and she had lost the plot altogether when Charlie arrived with the dreadful news. Her big brother Jack had been someone good and strong and true for her to look up to. A good role model and a reliable parent figure, unlike her two hopeless parents.

Whilst out of the mental hospital, on trial, Phyllis took Shirley for an outing to Henley Beach sometime in 1930. The little girl was delighted and held on tightly to her mummy's hand. She was frightened that her mother would disappear again and kept on looking up at her to make certain that she was happy and enjoying the outing. A heavy storm blew up and mother and child needed to shelter under the jetty for some time before it was safe to catch the tram back home again. Shirley snuggled her head into Phyllis's lap, squeezing her eyes tightly to shut out the stinging sand. Overhead she could hear the seagulls screeching and nearby the waves crashing onto the beach. Phyllis gently stroked her hair and sang a lullaby to her until the storm subsided. The bedraggled pair eventually dragged themselves through the sand and on towards the tram stop. Shirley could not stop smiling. Her mother had been nice to her.

Pinky Flat, a fair walk from their house, was another favourite outing and Shirley hid these memories away in her heart for all time as treasures to bring out and play with whenever she pined for her mother. Finally Phyllis broke down and was pronounced too ill and unstable to live alone. Charlie had had enough of her psychotic outbursts and refused to live with her anymore. Shirley was seen to be at risk even for day visits with her mother. Phyllis was returned for the last time to Parkside Mental Hospital and stayed there until two years before her death in October, 1962. The last two years of her life were spent in Northfield Mental Hospital, which was subsequently re-named Hillcrest Hospital in 1964, a decision which reflected the changing attitude to mental illness.

Someone to Watch Over Me

Shirley did not see her mother again until she was a mother herself, with seven children. When her last baby was born, she nervously visited her mother for Mother's Day. Her friend Gloria Purdie went with her for much needed moral support. Shirley was shaking as she walked into the hospital, a gift wrapped box of pretty blue slippers under her arm[1]. Phyllis too was shaking, but with excitement, as she puffed on her cigarette and joyfully spoke of her little girl Shirley who was coming to see her. Sadly she could not make the connection that little Shirley had grown into the woman standing before her. Shirley found this very distressing.

The staff had affectionately nick-named Phyllis 'Gilly' and seemed to be fond of their long-term patient. Also, some Christian women from Mile End Church of Christ had taken her under their wings and visited her, inviting her to their homes occasionally for Sunday lunch. She had a little dog in the hospital that one of them had kindly given her.

Sadly, Phyllis did not get to meet any of her grandchildren as they had been told that she had died when their mother was born.

---

[1] The author recalls seeing those blue satin slippers sitting in a box with tissue paper on the green laminex kitchen table. She was seventeen years old at the time and inquisitive. Such a sight was unusual in their home. She asked her mother who they were for? Her mother answered defensively "For your Grandmother." "But she has large feet. These are only a size five."

"For your other Grandmother, alright?"

The shock of this revelation was akin to a face slap and remembered for decades. She had always been told that her other Grandmother had died at Shirley's birth.

Years later, the author was regularly visiting Hillcrest Hospital with a group from her church. They sang and shared and then chatted over tea and biscuits with the residents. There were hugs and kisses and laughter. Phyllis was a resident at the time and she may have met one of the grandchildren after all.

Chapter Nine

"The true test of character is not how much we know what to do, but how we behave when we don't know what to do." John Holt

Charlie was an eternal optimist and he firmly believed that his sister would recover and that she and Shirley would be together once again. He had stayed on in the house on Henley Beach Road where Phyllis had lived with Shirley, paying the rent each week and visiting Phyllis at the hospital when he could, eagerly watching for her improvement. Sometimes he went the further distance and called on Flo and Percy so he could check up on his little niece.

He was angry with his brother-in-law for deserting Phyllis, but Percy was a charming bloke and Charlie was not one to hold grudges.

"Hello Percy."

"How are you Charlie?"

"How's the French polishing going? Heard you were starting up on your own."

"Yeah. I've had enough of working as a labourer. I'm renting a shop not far from you. The customers are starting to come in. Things are a bit tight everywhere though. Lucky I can sleep in the back room. Don't have to find extra rent money."

"Bet you're glad to be back at your trade."

"Too right. Call in sometime Charlie and I'll make you a cuppa. We can chew the fat like old times."

"Alright mate. I know where you are. I pass the group of shops with the horse and cart every day, out on my rounds."

Someone to Watch Over Me

"How's business going with you? Are you managing to keep your head above water?"

"Only just. I'm always robbing Peter to pay Paul, you know how it is. Bad times. So many people out of work. Reckon there's a depression not too far off. Anyway, we're laughing....people need to eat...... at least we still have work. Not like so many other poor sods."

"You're right old boy."

"Did you hear that Phyl will be out soon and Shirley will be able to be with her mother? I'm sure that Florrie will be relieved."

"You don't say? Getting better is she?"

"Yep. The doctor says that she's stable again. Really threw her when Jack died. The drugs they give her have calmed her down. She just needs a bit of rest to get over things and clear her head."

"Pigs will fly too, Charlie!"

Charlie steeled himself. He felt like taking a punch at his brother-in-law, but somehow controlled the urge. Flo was listening in on their conversation and butted in rudely.

"So you think Shirley will be able to go and live with you and Phyl, do you Charlie? Any idea how soon that will be?"

She didn't like Charlie and his scruffy clothes, but bought her green groceries from him now and then so that people would see what a good Christian woman she was.

They chatted about Shirley's future living arrangements and Charlie offered to take her with him, until Phyllis came home and settled back into her house. He explained that the social worker would call and check to make sure that everything was going well and Shirley was being looked after properly. Flo smiled sweetly, fluttering her eyelashes at Charlie in a flirtatious manner.

"Why Charlie, you sweet, sweet man. Do you mean it? You would be willing to take the child and care for her yourself until dear Phyl can? You are too good to be true. Did you hear that Percy? Your brother-in-law has offered to take Shirley in. Isn't

Someone to Watch Over Me

that wonderful? You will be able to carry on in your own business and not worry about her. She will be in good hands. When did you have in mind Charles?"

Charles William Thomas Carter had been abandoned himself as a child, charged with being a destitute child at ten years of age, and sent to the Industrial School in Magill. The Poor House.

He was a bachelor and unfamiliar with the needs of children, but a kind and generous man. He had fought, as a mere boy, to keep his family together, and now he was going to do the same for his sister's little family. He could read Flo like a book and knew that she did not like having a four year old around all of the time, cramping her style. He would do his best for this child, because no-one had rescued him as a lad and he knew what it felt like to be alone and frightened. He would learn to care for his little niece with the blind eye and the broken heart, until her own mother was well again.

It was settled.

Percy sighed deeply. Relief was written on his weary face. Freedom smelled good.

Flo caught his eye and smiled sweetly. She was much too old to be worrying about a little girl, especially one with a troubled past and a blind eye. Percy, in her opinion, needed to get on with his business and make a name for himself. He could pick up his responsibilities with Shirley later when he had some money and success behind him. She thought Charlie a bit of a loser, but that he had made the Gilfillans winners in this round.

Flo gave Charlie a sisterly hug and put the kettle on. It was time to celebrate.

Chapter Ten

"Happiness is different from pleasure. Happiness has something to do with struggling and enduring and accomplishing."
Jennifer Louden

She loved Uncle Charlie with her whole heart. He would take her with him on his rounds. They started at four a.m. It was hard to get out of bed, but if she didn't she would have to stay at home all day on her own.

Shirley remembered the time when she was four and she had been sick. Her uncle had told her that she would have to stay at home and care for herself as he had to do his rounds with his horse and cart and green groceries. She had tried to get out of bed, but had vomited and was shaking and weak. All through the night she had been hot and cold and thrashing about in her bed. Shirley let her head fall back onto her pillow and bit her lip to stop it trembling. As young as she was, she knew that her uncle felt very upset at having to leave her. There was no-one to call and she had to be brave.

He had harnessed Blackie and then popped back in to say goodbye and wish her well. He left a rag and bowl near her bed and kissed her on the forehead. She was hot and feverish. He went and fetched a mug of water and left that as well. Shrugging his shoulders, he walked out of the back door into the darkness of the morning. He heaved himself up on to his cart and clicked his tongue at Blackie who slowly plodded off out into the street. It would be a very long day, with no way of contacting his sick little niece or knowing if she was alright.

Sadly, this happened often as Shirley was a sickly child. Their diet was meagre because they were poor and there was no money for doctors or medicines. Some meals were missed and the two went hungry, with promises from Charlie for a grand meal tomorrow. Some days, no matter how sick she felt, Shirley would make herself get out of bed, dress and be ready to go on the cart. Anything would be better than to stay in the dark, lonely house all day on her own. There was no electricity, as they couldn't afford it. Instead, they had a kerosene lamp, which her uncle lit and placed in her room once he was up and dressed.

"What's for brekky?" she would ask.

"We have fried bacon and eggs and a sausage for my princess," he would tease as he scraped and buttered her toast.

"Just hurry along there my man," she would joke back and they would laugh together, devouring their meal of toast and a cup of tea.

The five year old hurriedly pulled on her woolly skirt and jumper. Her stockings were next and then her lace-up shoes. She had taken a while to learn how to tie her laces, but her uncle was very patient and she eventually caught on. He had been teaching her to do tomboy stitch with a wooden cotton reel and an old hair clip. He promised that when she mastered it, he would teach her to knit. She was so excited. She would knit a scarf for school. The other kids would see how clever she really was. On went her cap and she was ready for her breakfast and the day ahead.

They ate their breakfast quickly and then both drank their cup of tea. Uncle Charlie had made a fire in the front room grate when he arose and he made the toast over the coals while the kettle sang away over the heat. When they finished, Shirley turned around and around to warm herself until the very last moment, when her uncle doused the fire.

"We don't want to come home tired and hungry to find there is no home anymore because it has burned down."

"That would be terrible." Shirley quickly fetched her mug of water and poured that on the coals as well.

"Just to make sure that it is really out." She followed her uncle into her small room and watched him turn out the kerosene lamp and then they both walked to the back door, holding hands and walking in the blackness. Shirley popped quickly into the outside toilet, which Charlie called 'the dunny', and he waited outside for her because she was afraid in the dark. When she was ready, they hopped up onto the cart and set off to the market to buy the produce they would sell to their customers on their usual round.

"It's going to be a lovely day today Uncle Charlie. I just know it is. And we're going to make lots of nice money."

"I hope so little one. I sure hope so."

Chapter Eleven

"A child's eyes, those clear, wells of undefiled thought - what on earth can be more beautiful? Full of hope, love and curiosity, they meet your own. In prayer, how earnest, in joy, how sparkling, in sympathy, how tender!" Caroline Norton

It was good being a school girl. There were children to play with and things to learn. There were crayons to draw with and books to read. Lunch time meant games in the school yard. She loved skipping with the rope with a girl each end turning it. Her rhythm was faultless and she skipped better than most of her friends. It was her moment of triumph when she skipped the longest without tripping.

The worst part about school was the waiting after Uncle Charlie had left at five a.m. He had to trust her with the fire and the kerosene lamp. That was fine because she knew she could trust herself to get it right. It was the waiting on her own until the sun came up and knowing just when to take off for school that bothered her. She would sit on her bed watching out across the front veranda. When she saw the other kids heading off to school with their leather bags on their backs, Shirley would head off as well. Sometimes she walked with the other children. Sometimes their parents walked with them. Mostly she walked alone. She was short and her little legs could not keep up with the older boys and girls.

They were now living in Rankine Road, having moved from Phyllis's rental place on Henley Beach Road. It was such a long way. All the way from Rankine Road to the Thebarton Primary School, on South Road. Rain. Shine. She walked the distance there and back. Back to the empty house. Often she would go across the street and play with the children. Their family kept race-horses and the hay to feed them was stored in their shed. The children climbed and tumbled down the hay and played all sorts of imaginary games. They gathered some other children from along the road and they played street cricket some days. Shirley loved these days and hated the loneliness when the children had other things to do after school, or on week-ends.

Her favourite pastime of all was going to the pictures. This she did on her own, walking to the matinees at the Thebarton Picture Theatre on Saturday afternoons. Only on the days when there was money left over for such luxuries, though. Her Uncle had his interests on Saturday afternoons, and they included boxing, the races, or visiting his friends. Mainly she was home on her own and needed to make her own fun. When there was money for the movies she was so excited she could hardly sit still and wait. Her biggest challenge was knowing when to set off to walk the long distance to the theatre, on Henley Beach Road. The child mentioned her anxiety to Mrs Stock, her kindly neighbour, over the back fence one day, and her problem was solved.

"Shirley. Shirley. Come along dear, it's time to get going."

Shirley quickly skipped out of the back door and through the gate. She offered a friendly pat to Blackie and a thankful wave to Mrs. Stock as she skipped off happily. She was going to see a Shirley Temple film, 'Bright Eyes'.

"Thank you, I'll tell you about the picture later Mrs. Stock" she called " then you won't have to go but can save your pennies."

She skipped along the street holding on to the lump in her pocket through her grubby skirt, pretending to be like Shirley Temple, the actress who was three years younger and also as cute as a button. Uncle Charlie had tied the money into a corner of his handkerchief and she did not want to lose it. There was no more where that came from, and she would have to wait for sometime before there was money for her to go to the pictures again.

Shirley noticed how the other children in the street loved staying home and having a "sickie." Longingly she noticed how their mothers fussed over them, tucking them into their nice cosy beds, bringing them drinks, sponging and feeding them special 'beef tea', taking their temperatures, and reading them stories. When Shirley was ill and needing to stay home she was completely alone, all day. There was no-one to hold her head when she vomited and no-one to empty her bowl and bring her a refreshing drink. Except for one day, when she had mumps. Shirley was lying in bed, her face swollen and sore, and feeling very sick and sorry for herself. It was deathly quiet in the house. She heard the back door open and someone step inside. She was terrified. No-one ever called on a work day. She dragged herself out of bed and got on her tummy and slid under the bed to hide from the intruder. Her heart was pounding in her chest and she tugged at the blanket hanging over the edge of the mattress, pulling it down a little to hide her.

Footsteps approached, through the kitchen and then to her bedroom door. She dare not breathe. The intruder walked slowly over to the bed and stood there. The blanket was pulled back up onto the bed and Shirley suddenly saw two eyes peering at her.

"What are you doing here lass? Come on out so I can get a good look at you."

Shirley was trembling and felt even worse. "You look awful child. I am sorry to have scared you. I should have called out. I thought you might be sleeping. Looks to me like you have a good case of the mumps. You have a face like the moon right now. Let's see what we can do to make you more comfortable."

Mrs. Bennett, their kind neighbour, had heard that Shirley was at home and feeling poorly. One of the parents of one of the local children had mentioned the fact. It had bothered her all day that the child was on her own without any nurturing and she

Someone to Watch Over Me

finally decided to visit. She had a feeling that Charlie probably left his door open all day, like most of their neighbours, and she was correct.

As Shirley slowly lay down on her bed she noticed that Mrs. Bennett had a piece of flannel, torn from an old garment in her hand. She frowned as she wondered what it was for.

"Don't worry lassie. I have soaked this piece of flannel that used to be part of Mr. Bennett's shirt, in some hot salty water. We'll wrap it around your poor face and it should make you feel much better."

She did feel better, but more because of the kindness of her neighbour than the healing properties of the salty flannel.

Her Uncle Charlie worried about her a great deal. He had no idea how to care for a sick little girl. He kept hoping that Phyllis would get well enough to come to live with him and his little niece. He had visited her in 'Parkside' recently and she had been awful to him. She had been out of control and very abusive. She had accused him of trying to punch her body with his words, from miles away. He thought that the least she could do was to be grateful for all he was doing and sacrificing to look after her daughter. Instead, she accused and abused and yelled. He left feeling like a dog that had been kicked by its owner. He loved Phyl and he was hurt. It would be a long time before he visited her again.

Whenever Shirley became seriously ill, her uncle took her to the Adelaide Children's Hospital in North Adelaide. She stayed there a number of times, and loved the clean, crisp sheets, the food and special drinks, but only some of the nurses. The mean ones scared her and when Uncle Charlie came to visit he brought the comics page from "The Sunday Mail" to cheer her up. She loved him reading Ginger Meggs and he always managed to get her to smile.

On one occasion, while she was staying in the hospital, she felt sick and very thirsty. She asked for a drink but the nurse was

Someone to Watch Over Me

busy and crabby. She was unkind to Shirley and snapped at her crossly. The little girl started crying for her uncle.

"Charlie, Charlie. I want Charlie," she cried over and over again. She screamed and sobbed into her pillow for him. No-one came to comfort her. She was out on the veranda, with some other children, because the wards were over-crowded. The other children had books and stuffed toys. Shirley had nothing to cuddle for comfort. All she wanted was Charlie, as he always managed to cheer her up and make her feel better. He was her family now. Eventually the nurse came and gave her a drink of water from the water bag which hung from a hook on the veranda. Charlie never came. He was working.

When she finally returned home with her uncle, she had a lot to tell him about her stay in hospital, and chatted on and on, telling him the good and bad experiences.

"Did you make any special friends?" asked her uncle.

"Yes I did. Her name is Mavis. She is my best friend. We were like sisters. We would get into bed together and talk and laugh and read books. We were sad to say goodbye and we cried and cried. Her mummy came to pick her up. She was a lovely mummy. She gave me a present."

Shirley proudly held up a book for Charlie to see.

"I want you to read it to me every night before I go to sleep. I will sleep with it under my pillow every night too."

Shirley stopped the chatter and sadness seemed to swirl around them like an early morning mist.

"Mavis is so lucky," whispered the child.

Charlie could see that his niece was pining for a mother she had never had. A gentle mother with a soft touch and loving words. A mother to feel safe with, who comforted and encouraged and sang. He pulled her onto his knee. He started to sing to her. He had a pleasant enough voice and they had a special song which he sang to her at times like these. A song that she remembered for the rest of her days.

Someone to Watch Over Me

"There's no-one like mother to me
No matter how cross she may be -
My heart overflows with the beautiful thought
For there's no-one like mother to me."

Chapter Twelve

"If you bungle raising your children, I don't think whatever else you do matters very much." Jackie Kennedy Onassis

Shirley was inconsolable. She was curled up tightly, hugging her battered, smelly old pillow. She had been like this for the past hour. Charlie was shattered. He knew that she would take it badly, but didn't expect her to be this upset.

The child was gulping and hiccupping and her body heaved and fell as she convulsed, while crying as if her heart would break in two. A couple of times she was quiet and he thought it was over. But she would start up again, sobbing uncontrollably and it was breaking his heart. Guilt settled around his shoulders like a heavy, serge cloak.

He had tried to reason with her. He tried to bribe her with the promise of the Saturday matinee. He offered a visit to her father and her grandmother. Nothing cheered her because the one thing she wanted was being pulled away from her. She would never get it back. They couldn't be partners anymore. He needed to move on with his life and his young side-kick, for the past five years, was not part of his future plans.

Daisy May Bates had captured his sense of adventure. She was an amazing woman, living in a tent at seventy five years of age, and working as a welfare worker amongst the Australian Aborigines. She spent her time rescuing them, helping them and preaching their cause. Her base was somewhere near Oodea, in the north of South Australia. Camping with meagre creature comforts, Daisy dressed each day, in spite of the soaring temperatures, in her preferred Victorian, up to the neck fashions and worked hard to help the people about whom she was passionate. She lived free from the entrapments of society and coped without the things that were a necessity for city dwellers. She was not defined by what she had, but by what she did for her fellow man.

Daisy Bates wrote and delivered her lectures with great enthusiasm. She was truly inspiring and eventually on the first of January, 1934, she was appointed a Commander of the Order of the British Empire for her work amongst aborigines. Her award was mentioned in 'The Advertiser' along with the venue and times for her meetings in Adelaide. Charlie went along to hear what she had to say and stayed around to talk with her after the formalities were over. He was fascinated with this woman who was mother to so many. Her heart was so large and she cared so much. Unlike his own mother who cared so little for her own children, and so much for 'the bottle.' He wanted to spend more time with Daisy and learn more about the work she was doing. He invited her around to his house to chat further. Her vision, her motivation, her enthusiasm for her cause inspired him. He wanted to make a change to the direction his life had taken. He was forty nine, for Pete's sake. He wanted a flag to ride under - like his brother Jack, the brave Light Horseman. He wanted to be a hero. He wanted a cause to believe in. He wanted his life to count.

He closed his mind to the truth that he was all of those things to a sadly deserted nine year old. His green grocery round was sold for a pittance. A little girl's heart was broken yet again.

Chapter Thirteen

"Every instance of heartbreak can teach us powerful lessons about creating the kind of love we really want." Martha Beck

They stood together at the wooden door. Both with shoulders stooped. Holding hands and eyes fixed on the large, heavy and round door knocker.

He put down the old battered case and knocked three times, willing no-one to answer. He now saw with clarity how very much his little niece had come to mean to him. He had rescued her from abuse and she had rescued him right back from loneliness and despair. They had spent five years of poverty and deprivation together - hard years that had been softened by their affection and caring for each other. She had become the child he had never had. He had become the mother and father that she wished she had.

"Be brave 'little flea.' You will be part of a big family now. You will have lots of mummies. Lots of brothers and sisters. Good food. Warm clothes. Toys and books. Nice outings. You'll see. You'll love it." He had said these things to her many times in the last few days. Now he was trying to convince himself that they were true.

"I'll visit you whenever I can. But I have to go up north to help the aborigines. You don't want me to let them down do you? There's lots of boys and girls up there who need my help."

"But I need you. I could come too and help you. I wouldn't be any trouble. I promise."

She started to cry and he squatted down and hugged her in his big teddy-bear arms. The door opened. Charlie jumped to his feet and his heart pounded in his chest. Shirley started to shake all over. She held on to his hand with both of hers in a vice-like grip.

The red brick building was unattractive and unwelcoming. The door was plain and unfriendly. The woman who it opened to was all of these things and worse. Her dress was black and down to the ground and she had a strange black thing on her head, with a white tight-looking head band. Around her waist was a rope and hanging off it was a very large cross with a little man hanging on it. Shirley had seen a crucifix before, but not on someone's belt. The woman did not smile. In fact, she frowned and acted impatiently as if she had been interrupted and was cross.

She doesn't look like anyone's nice mummy to me, went screaming through Shirley's mind and she turned on her heels and started to run away. But Charlie was expecting her to try to escape and he quickly caught her.

"Now that was a stupid thing to do child. You should be grateful that we have found a place for you here. We are full up and can't take everyone that comes to our door. Anyway, you've come at a busy time, so say goodbye to your uncle, girl. We must get you bathed and settled in."

Her voice was sharp and menacing.

"Can't he come in?" she whispered, her voice breaking.

"No. It's best he just goes. Say goodbye, and hurry along. I don't have all day you know."

Charlie was starting to have second thoughts. This was not how he had imagined saying goodbye to her. The nun seemed mean. He cheered himself up with the thought that she was only one of many and must be in a bad mood. So many children would make even a saint bad-tempered some days.

He knelt down and Shirley threw her arms around his neck, sobbing and pleading into his collar. He knew her courage and had seen it displayed over and over again. He knew that she would deal with this and survive, no matter what was ahead for her.

"We will always be partners, little flea. I'll be back. This is only for a little while. Be brave. You're my little soldier, remember. You can do anything if you make up your mind to."

The nun backed into the darkness, dragging the sad little girl by the arm as she went. Charlie quickly picked up her tiny case and placed it inside the doorway as the door closed with a loud bang.

It closed on his little niece's screams and pleas. His child for five years. More than half of her life.

He was frozen to the spot. Their parting left an indelible impression on his mind forever. The pain of relinquishing her would remain part of his every day. His face wet with tears, he stood fighting the urge to tear down the door and rescue her back from whatever was ahead.

Chapter Fourteen

"A thousand words will not leave so deep an impression as one deed." Henrik Ibsen

After her initial shock at moving into an orphanage, Shirley started to analyse her new living conditions. She worked out very quickly that all the children were unhappy, hungry, bored and scared. The cause of their fear was the women who were in charge of them. All dressed like bats in their ugly black outfits, and most of them were nasty and mean. A couple of the older girls quickly took her aside and warned her about the ones to be especially wary of, and of the idiosyncrasies of each woman.

Sister Francesca was one of the nastiest of all and would pinch the children without warning, often during morning prayers which were held daily at 6 a.m. The girls were made to kneel on the hard wooden floor in their nightgowns, in the centre of the huge dormitory. It was so cold in winter and so uncomfortable. Were they to move ever so slightly, or complain at all, they were in big trouble. Those pinches were not easily forgotten.

Sister Germaine was fastidious about no drinks before early communion which was held every morning at 7 am in the church. Some of the girls would wake up thirsty, but were not allowed to cup their hands for a drink at the basin in their dormitory, or to open their mouths for a few drops of water under the shower. Apparently God deemed this unforgivable. Sister Germaine threatened hellfire in the hereafter and hell here on earth to any defiant child who would dare to disobey her unwritten law. The brave who defied her when she was looking away were held in high esteem for their courage.

Sister Angelina was very cross with the little ones who wet their cot mattresses. She made them carry the wet, smelly little mattresses around on their backs all morning. The older girls were made to tie the mattresses across the shoulders of the little bed wetters. The tiny children hated it and cried and squirmed and protested, but this did not cause the nun to take pity on them. Her intention was to shame them into dry nights. It didn't seem to occur to her (or most of the nuns for that matter) that the children may not yet have control over their bladders at this young age. Nor did it seem to occur to them that they were missing their families, living in a strange place and emotionally distraught. Shirley wanted to rescue the children, but was quickly warned not to do so, or she would be severely punished.

Sister Marguerite-Marie was like a sergeant major, inspecting the girls each night in their beds, ensuring their hands were outside of the covers and crossed over their chests. This sleeping position was mandatory and also supervised. Each of the girls had to lie on their backs, as if in a coffin. Shirley had no idea what this was all about, but got the giggles when it was explained to her in whispers. Apparently, it was disgusting to touch yourself in certain places. This act made you a very bad girl, sent you to hell and made God very angry with you indeed. It also turned Sister Marguerite-Marie into a fire-eating dragon.

Sister Dorcas was in charge of the sewing and was not nice at all. She taught heavenly fancy work and heaven help you if you made a mistake or did not pay attention. She was impatient, critical and nasty with her students. No matter how well a girl may sew, this sister was never guilty of giving praise. The girls had a few choice names for her. They would make up new ones and try to outdo each other to see who was the most creative. They would wait until they were alone and then share them and laugh until the tears ran down their cheeks. Shirley liked the name she made up, "Sister Snip 'n Snap" best of all.

Sister Beatrice was in charge of the kitchen. Everyone wanted to keep on her good side, because if they managed to get kitchen duties, they just might get a few extra scraps to eat. The children were always hungry. Treats like jam or treacle were foreign to them. Not to the priest however. Treacle was reserved for the nuns and the priest, whenever he visited St. Joseph's at Largs Bay. He, of course, did not like his crusts. These offensive pieces of food were kindly cut off for him, and the lucky children who happened to be working in the kitchen at the time, scrambled to get them. The child kitchen hands learned to spread the treacle carefully to the edges for the priest.

On the other hand, kitchen duty meant hard work. Long days. Heavy manual work. Large bags of flour and sugar had to be dragged up the steep stairs from the cellar which was also the home to a number of large, mean-looking rats. It meant being yelled at, ridiculed when you did something wrong, and endless exacting work that was designed for adults, not small children.

Sister Columbo was in charge of the laundry. It was an outside laundry with an unending pile of washing to be done. She was always in a bad mood. In fact, according to the older girls, her mood had not changed for years. It did not matter how hard you tried to do the right thing with the mountains of clothes, towels, sheets, bedspreads and blankets, you always did it wrong and were too slow. "You stupid girl" was her catch phrase. She usually accompanied it with a sharp slap, if she could reach the shameful offender. Everyone hated laundry duty. The washing was too heavy for the children, but they had to do it anyway. Sister Columbo had no mercy when accidents happened, as invariably they did. Everyone was wary of the mangle. The children called it "The Gobbler." It chewed up victims who were momentarily distracted. Shirley became a victim and her sad encounter left her scarred for life.

Someone to Watch Over Me

Sister Cecilia was the youngest and the sweetest. The girls looked out for fallen bobby pins from the other nuns to give to her, as she was their favourite. She was gentle with the children when she was alone with them, but conformed to the expectations of the older nuns when they were around. Sadly, she looked away when they were severe with their punishments, or harsh with their words.

Sister Charlotte was the school teacher. Anyone could see she was a poor choice for the job. The classroom was just one of the rooms in the orphanage. It was bare, colourless and uninviting. Laughter was never heard in this room. The nun made fun of the boys and girls, in a mean and sarcastic way. Ridicule was her middle name. You gave her the answer she wanted, or suffered the consequences. Shirley had missed out on a lot of time at school whilst staying with Charlie. Because they had no books in their house, she had not learned to read very well. There was no doubt that she had difficulty with literacy and numeracy because she possibly had a dash or more of dyslexia. Shirley had never made friends with words or numbers and would struggle throughout her life with them.

Meanwhile, she struggled in St. Joseph's school room. Sister Charlotte fumed. "You dumb cluck!" she screamed. "A small child would know that."

The other children sat motionless. They were secretly glad that it was not them copping it this time.

"You stupid, stupid girl. You are an idiot. Get out of my classroom and stay out. You can spend your time in the kitchen from now on. Sister Beatrice needs a permanent kitchen hand. She can put up with you. Peeling potatoes is all you're good for. Don't you dare come back here again!"

Shirley was devastated. She loved to learn and was hungry to improve her reading skills. She also wanted to be with the other children. Learning together. Spending time together. Instead, she was banished to the kitchen, where she spent the rest of her time at St. Josephs.

Sister Gertrude was the nun to fear the most. She was extremely nasty. She was mean like a snarling dog. She had a heart made of stone. Her punishments were vindictive, cruel and demeaning. She claimed she did it for the good of the children at all times. She was "answerable to her God to make good girls out of her charges." Sometimes just the threat of a beating made the girls cower and obey her. Other times her victims wore the welts that she beat into their tender bodies with her infamous belt. Her arm would be raised high above her head, her other hand holding the arm of the offending child. She put her whole self into the execution of her God-given duty. "In the name of the Father (swish) the Son (swish) and the Holy Spirit (swish)."

The worst of her punishment was isolation. Shirley was to be a victim of this horror. She would never entirely recover.

"Charlie. Please come and get me. Dear God, I promise to be a good girl, always. Please send Charlie to get me and take me home. Please make him come back from up north. Please. Dear Mary, Mother of God. Please. I can't stay here any longer."

Her three friends were sisters. They slept near Shirley and heard her crying and praying.

"Shh! Shirley. Shh!! She'll hear you."

They had lived here for years and looked out for their new little friend. Rita was now her best friend and she was worried about the repercussions for Shirley should the nun overhear her prayers.

Too late! Sister Marguerite-Marie rushed over to her bed breathing fire.

"Why you ungrateful little wretch. You wicked child. After all we do for you. Day in and day out. Putting ourselves out for you good-for-nothings. Tomorrow you'll scrub the entire dormitory floor. On your own. And you'd better do it well, or you'll do it again."

Someone to Watch Over Me

Shirley assumed the correct sleeping position, but sleep did not come and rescue her for some time.

She cried quietly, the tears running down her face and wetting the pillow. She did not pray this time. She was a bad girl and Jesus must not like her.

Chapter Fifteen

"Chance is always powerful. Let your hook be always cast; in the pool where you least expect it, there will be a fish."   Ovid Taylor

Shirley had been kneeling on the hard wooden floor for two long hours now and her knees were very sore. She was scrubbing the huge dormitory floor with a scrubbing brush and a bucket of soapy water. She had nothing to kneel on and a few rags to wipe up the floor as she went.

The other children had been in the school room most of the morning, but one of her friends, Gloria, had managed to sneak in, on the way to the toilet, to see how she was going.

Usually there were several children at once scrubbing the floor, because it was a very large room. Shirley was being punished by a spiteful woman and made to do it alone. She was hurting all over. Especially her poor knees. She was getting very tired. She stood up to stretch herself and see how much more she had to do. To her dismay, she wasn't even half way through.

The water in the metal bucket had become very dirty and she needed some more fresh rags for mopping up. She placed the scrubbing brush and messy rags together at the edge of the room and headed for the outside troughs to empty the bucket and run fresh water into it. She would continue working with cold water and no soap because she was too scared to ask for anything from the crabby nun.

Someone to Watch Over Me

Sister Marguerite-Marie said that she could have nothing to eat or drink until the job was completed to her satisfaction. Shirley was thirsty and hungry from the sheer physical effort. She dare not ask for anything, though, for fear of further punishment. Next time she might get a beating like poor Anna did.

Just two days earlier, her friend Anna, Jacinta's sister, had asked for something more to eat as the watered down tuna stew had left her feeling hungry. Sister Germaine had blown up like a poisonous puffer fish, and yelled at Anna in a raging temper. Anna had a temper too and yelled back.

"I only asked for more food 'cos I was hungry. All us kids hate that runny horrid tuna stew and we eat it 'cos there's nothing else. It doesn't fill us up much and we won't get anything else 'til breakfast."

The children froze. No-one spoke. They sensed that Anna's bravery was going to cost her dearly.

Anna stood her ground with her hands on her hips, looking the nun in the eyes. Eyes that were now wild like that of a mad horse. The nun flew at her, grabbing one of her arms she half dragged her into another room. The room where the belt was kept. Some of the children put their hands over their ears so they would not hear Anna's screams. They still heard them though and were deeply affected by the eleven year-old's cries of pain and injustice. Every child present decided that asking for extra food was something they would never do.

Shirley kept on scrubbing the floor. Sister Marguerite-Marie came and checked on her progress once or twice and made her go back over a couple of spots that were not scrubbed to her satisfaction.

Lunch-time came and Shirley was not allowed to leave her chore until Sister said so. She was starving now and very thirsty. Sister Cecilia approached the bullying sister gingerly and pointed out that if only she could have something to eat and drink,

Shirley would get the job completed faster. Sister Marguerite-Marie was sullen and determined.

"Not a morsel until she has finished the whole floor!"

She stood her ground with her nose in the air and her arms folded sternly on her bosom, her face made of stone.

Sister Cecilia looked at the nine-year old, who was trying to relieve her reddened knees of their pain by moving them from one position to another. She was now squatting on her haunches while she scrubbed, obviously in great discomfort. The lass did this for a few minutes and then went back on her knees again, sliding back when she had scrubbed along the long length of the dormitory.

Suddenly Shirley burst into tears and cried out in pain. Sister Cecilia rushed to her to see what the matter was. The child pointed to her knee. Sister Cecilia could see that both knees had been rubbed raw. Now she had a huge splinter from the old floorboards that had imbedded itself in the raw part of her right knee. Sister Marguerite-Marie came hurriedly to see what all the fuss was about. The younger, kinder nun asked for the child to be relieved of the rest of the scrubbing because she was now injured and needed the splinter attended to. She pointed out the skin had been rubbed from both of her knees and they were raw and sore. The older nun would not back down. The girl would see out her punishment and receive no reprieve. This would be a lesson to her in the future to obey the God-given rules and would make a better girl of her. Sister Cecilia had done her best and she patted Shirley on the shoulder for moral support and sadly returned to her duties.

Eventually Shirley completed her task, somehow twisting her little body into all sorts of positions so as to avoid kneeling. No-one ever thought to remove the large splinter and this proved to be a very dangerous oversight. Next morning Shirley was too weak and sore to get up and was allowed to miss early morning

Someone to Watch Over Me

prayers and communion. She also missed breakfast and felt worse and worse as the day started to fade into night.

She stayed in bed the next day and could not eat anything. The following day she was sent bread and milk, consisting of stale bread broken up into pieces in a bowl and swamped with milk. She tried to eat but felt far too sick. She remained on her bed all day for several days. No-one came near her and she was very scared. She knew that she was ill and should see a doctor. Her leg was hot and painful and throbbing. When the girls came in at the end of the day she could hardly bear the noise.

One of the girls kept telling the sister just how sick Shirley was and how thin she had become. The sister eventually had a closer look at the child and quickly rushed off to call a doctor. He came urgently and examined her on her bed, because she was too ill to move. Dr. McIntosh was a pleasant young doctor, dressed in a grey suit, white shirt and blue tie. His suit looked like it had seen better days and his shirt was crumpled and stained. He was more interested in the welfare of his patients than his appearance and hurried to Shirley's bedside to examine her. When he lifted the grey blanket and took one look at her injured leg he swore under his breath. He felt her forehead, which was burning up. He quickly swept Shirley up in his arms. He was too angry with the nuns to speak to any of them. He carried the sick little girl straight out to his car, laying her down on the back seat. He drove her hurriedly to the Children's Hospital in North Adelaide.

Shirley was taken immediately into the operating room and her poisoned knee was lanced and the ugly splinter removed. Pus and blood gushed out. Her knee was tenderly dressed and she was transported on a bed with wheels into a fresh and welcoming ward. She stayed in the hospital for a week, and under Dr. McIntosh's instructions, she was given penicillin to fight off the infection in her body, and good food to build her up again. She had become de-hydrated in the orphanage and he ordered an enticing variety of drinks, including flat lemonade to re-hydrate her.

The kindly doctor did not want her to return immediately to St. Joseph's Orphanage, so he organised for her to go to Mt. Lofty Home for Convalescents. It took her a further week to regain her strength and sparkle. She loved it at the lovely home that was an annex of the Children's Hospital. There were always a great line of slippers in the hallway. The floors were highly polished and no-one was allowed to wear their shoes inside. It was like a palace to the little girl who had never seen anything so grand.

Shirley went black-berrying with the other children, picking the fat, juicy blackberries from the thorny bushes. They had to be very careful not to be scratched by the sharp thorns. Their reward was a delicious dessert of scrumptious berries, sprinkled with a little sugar. The recovering children played happily together in the beautiful gardens. There were toys and books and people to play with. Shirley had a taste of heaven and dreaded going back to hell.

Someone to Watch Over Me

Chapter Sixteen

"Expect the best. Prepare for the worst. Capitalise on what comes." Zig Ziglar

"Is she looking?" Shirley was outside in the yard with the other girls and boys and they had just finished playing a casual form of basketball with Sister Charlotte. It was a Saturday.

They were now free to make their own fun. They would be outside until tea-time and Shirley was hungry. She was also hot. Running around in the itchy woollen dress had heated her body and she had nothing to take off to cool down. She had grabbed the dress from the laundry basket this morning, trying to get in the front of the line. If you were down the line, you had to take the dregs. It didn't seem to matter if something fitted or not. Shirley's dress was ugly and it was far too big. The dress was the least of her problems at the moment. She was hungry and couldn't keep her eyes off the fat, juicy, red berries on the bushes that ran alongside the fence and adjacent to the netball court

"No, she isn't looking. She has her back to us talking with Bobby. You better be quick though."

Jacinta was her look-out. Shirley quickly grabbed a handful of berries and stuffed them into her pocket.

"Am I still safe?"

The scavenger wanted to gather more for her friend.

"Yep, but you better be quick. Looks like she's moving away."

The plucky youngster grabbed another handful and stuffed them into her other pocket. She took Jacinta's hand and walked her around the side of the building, out of the view of the nun in charge. They giggled with glee at their wickedness and quickly devoured the berries, making certain that there was no tell-tale juice to be seen.

Tea was usually a sandwich, except on Friday nights, and it was never enough. Runny tuna stew was the "Friday night special" and hated by all.

The children loved visitor's day and Shirley discovered early on, that raiding the bins was a favourite past-time after the visitors left. Some brought oranges, or bananas or apples. The residents of St. Joseph's children's 'prison' rarely received treats like fresh fruit and made the most of eating the skins of bananas and oranges and also the cores of apples, finding them like exquisite treasures, discarded in the bins. They licked their lips savouring the taste of these fruits in the skins.

Bobby was one of the younger children and a favourite of Shirley's. She often tried to obtain extra morsels of food for him. He would cry with hunger when his stomach ached from emptiness. She would cheer him with a piece of food sneaked out of the kitchen in one of her pockets. He had been told by Sister Gertrude that he could not make his first communion until he stopped sucking his two middle fingers. It annoyed the nasty woman who saw his comfort mechanism as a dreadful sin. In Catholic philosophy, as interpreted by the bitter and twisted nuns in St. Joseph's, this finger sucking condemned him to hell as he wasn't made acceptable until he had taken "the body and blood of Christ." What an awful God those disturbed nuns believed in. Praise the blessed name of Jesus that He is nothing like the image they portrayed.

Better still than visitors' day were the week-ends when some of the children went to stay with kindly couples or families. Everyone hoped that they would be chosen and they put on their best smiles and manners, wishing they could put on best clothes as well. Jacinta, Anna and Muriel, three sisters, all looked out for

Someone to Watch Over Me

each other and now included Shirley in their family circle, looking out for her as well. The girls had chosen a nicer looking skirt and almost matching jumper for her from the clean laundry basket, and had helped her to comb her hair. The ten year old had plaits when she arrived one year ago at St. Joseph's Orphanage. They had been unceremoniously chopped off by Sister Gertrude, and thrown into the bin like some piece of unwanted rubbish. Shirley had been horrified and had to fight the urge to rush and rescue them. Her hair had not even been tidied up, but just left ragged by the huge scissors.

Her clothes did not fit too badly today, really, and her socks and lace-up shoes looked alright, so she began to keenly hope that she would be chosen to visit with someone. She smoothed out her crumpled forest green skirt that had once had pleats which sadly disappeared many washes ago. Her pale pink jumper didn't look too bad with the green skirt and her spirits lifted.

Sadly, she missed out again and watched with tears of disappointment as Barbara with the pretty face and beautiful eyes walked hand in hand with the happy older couple to their stately car. Two of the boys went with a younger couple with no children and they were enjoying themselves on the way to the couple's old Ford as the man ruffled up their hair and laughed with them about something.

It seemed to Shirley that she was just too old to be chosen. All those that went on visits seemed to be younger children.

But, all good things come to those who wait, and Shirley was eventually picked for a home visit with a young couple who were childless. They were beautiful, their house was beautiful, their golden dog was beautiful and their food was beautiful. Shirley's heart was glowing with sheer joy. The kindly couple felt sorry for Shirley in her ugly clothes and took her to a shop and bought her a magnificent emerald green velvet dress with a pretty cape. She was a film-star. Shirley Temple! She slept in a comfortable bed with a pretty lace cover and there was a dressing table with a mirror. There were pretty ballet pictures on the walls. At the windows were flimsy white curtains which floated in the breeze from the open windows. She had a wardrobe. She hung the dreadful clothes in it and wore the velvet dress all week-end. They had pretty little pink pyjamas with rose buds for her to wear, with matching pink slippers. She had a warm, soapy bath and then put on her pyjamas, pretending to be a normal little girl.

After tea time and her bath, Mrs. Wilson sat at the piano and started playing some popular songs and they all ended up singing. When they forgot the words Mr. Wilson made up words to fill the gaps and they all ended up laughing. Mr. and Mrs. Wilson complimented her on her lovely voice and encouraged her to sing a song she knew, on her own. She was shy and looked down at her shoes. Mrs. Wilson started playing a song that came out in February 1935 and was very popular with everyone.

"Here is a lovely song that your namesake sings, Shirley. Join in when you like. I feel sure you will know this one."

Shirley's eyes brightened as she remembered hearing this song played on the radio at the Mt. Lofty Home for Convalescents. She and the nurses and the children would sing along with it and it was loved by all of them.

"On the Good Ship Lollipop,"[2] played Mrs. Wilson, singing out the words as she played.

Shirley lifted her head and a burst of pride rushed through her as she sang out strongly. Her new friends the Wilsons smiled as she sang, nodding their heads with approval. How happy she felt to have her singing appreciated so warmly. She would never ever forget this wonderful moment.

Sleeping in her bed was like sleeping on a cloud. It was the first time she had slept on such a bed or in such a lovely room. She wanted to stay awake just to enjoy the experience. She thought of the horrid lumpy ticking mattresses in St. Jo's and the

---

[2] From the movie, "Bright Eyes." Composed by Richard A. Whiting and Lyrics by Sydney Clare.

Someone to Watch Over Me

rusty iron bases which the children were made to de-bug regularly with bobby pins.

No bugs in this place, thought Shirley. *Wish I could always live here.* She let herself hope.

All too soon Mr. Wilson had the car out the front, ready to transport her all the way back from Forestville to Largs Bay. A very long distance. Shirley did not want the journey to end and loved looking out the window as the houses whizzed past. She admired the gardens, a lovely contrast of colour to her experience in the home at Largs Bay, and she looked longingly at the children playing in their well kept front yards.

"If only........." she sighed.

Kindly Mrs. Wilson had allowed her to wear her beautiful new dress and cape back to St. Joseph's and she could hardly wait for her friends to see how pretty she looked. The velvet looked like something a princess would wear as the light caught it and Shirley absolutely loved it. The Wilsons smiled with pleasure as they saw her joy and kissed her goodbye when it was time for their departure. Shirley hugged them both and thanked them over and over again for a wonderful weekend and such a beautiful dress and pretty pyjamas and matching slippers. The ten year old's face was a picture of happiness and love. She watched as her new friends waved goodbye, blowing kisses at them.

The moment the Wilsons were out of sight, Sister Gertrude flew at Shirley and forced up her arms, yanking the gorgeous dress up over her head.

"Pride cometh before a fall young girl," she quoted. "We want no conceited little brats in our home!"

She turned on her heel with the lovely dress and cape, pyjamas and slippers all tucked possessively under her arm. Shirley watched them disappear through the doorway, standing there in her singlet and panties. Stripped of her pleasure in an instant, tears of disappointment and injustice flowed freely. She never saw her treasures again.

Someone to Watch Over Me

Chapter Seventeen

'Distrust all in whom the impulse to punish is powerful'
Friedrich Nietzsche

Shirley watched out each weekend for the Wilsons, sure that they would come for her again. She fussed over her appearance, trying to look her best. One day one of her friends managed to get hold of a bit of ribbon and Jacinta tied it under Shirley's hair, fastening it into a bow on top. She felt pretty and hoped so much that the beautiful young couple with no children would return for her. They never did.

Shirley determined to find them. She knew that they had liked her. They had been so nice to her and they all had such a lovely time. She had felt accepted by them. They treated her as if she was someone special and normal and nice. She had opened like a bud to the sun, basking in their loving kindness. She wanted to feel like that again. She would remember the way to their house. She had watched with great interest on the trip to their place on that beautiful weekend of her dreams.

The clever little girl waited until the coast was clear. Once again Jacinta was her ally and told her when it was safe to go, looking out across the yard towards the gates.

"No nuns in sight. Are you sure you want to do this? If they catch you they'll kill you. You know what they say about anyone trying to escape."

Jacinta was scared for her best friend, but excited at the same time.

Someone to Watch Over Me

"I must find them, they may want to adopt me. They can't have kids. I heard them talking about it. I think they liked me. They loved me singing. We could be a happy family."

Shirley had a dream and nothing would stop her.

Jacinta checked from the window again and gave Shirley a quick nod.

"Go now," she said urgently. "Run as fast as you can and good luck."

The runaway hurried through the door, across the yard and out through the gate. Her heart was beating fast and her head felt strange with the excitement. It was a wonderful sense of freedom. It was also scary. She looked behind and no-one was coming after her. She ran faster. She ran and ran and ran until she was completely exhausted and had to stop for a minute. She quickly looked back where she had come from and saw that she had come a long way and still no-one was chasing her. This encouraged her no end and she took off again, turning into the road that the Wilsons had taken.

She had been walking for hours and was no longer certain that she was on the right road. The sun was starting to set and it would be getting dark before too long. It was getting very cold as the night air set in and she pulled her cardigan together to keep out the chill. She picked up her feet and ploughed on steadfastly in the general direction of Forestville, a distance of some eighteen kilometres away.

Hunger and thirst were bothering her, but she had learned over the years, through difficult and deprived circumstances, to push down these yearnings and think about something else. She made herself think about the Wilsons. She had sung Uncle Charlie's song "There's no-one like mother to me....." and Mrs. Wilson had picked out the tune on her piano and sung it with her. Mrs. Wilson had blown her nose and said she was getting a cold, but Shirley didn't believe her. She could tell that she had tears in her eyes. She must have been sad about having no children.

Someone to Watch Over Me

    Shirley's feet were hurting now, but she kept on because it was dark and she would need to find somewhere to sleep overnight. She thought of her friends back at St. Joseph's and wondered if they had all managed to keep her secret about her escape. They would be getting ready for bed now and whispering amongst themselves. She knew that many of the girls in her dormitory would be aware that she was missing and some would be imagining all sorts of reasons for her absence. Most would never imagine that she was brave enough to run away because the sisters threatened very harsh punishment indeed for anyone who attempted escape.

    Shirley was confused. She had come to a crossroads and she didn't know which direction to take. She started out, and then hesitated and changed direction. She stopped in her tracks and decided to go back to her first choice. She was confused. It was getting dark. There was a light on in the window of a friendly and warm looking house and she argued with herself for a few minutes. Finally the child decided to knock on the door and ask for directions. She was invited in by the nice lady of the house, who seemed surprised to find a young girl at her door at nine o'clock at night. No questions were asked, but Shirley was offered a warm drink of chocolate and a piece of fruit from a pretty fruit bowl. Further food was offered and she was invited to sit at their table with the lace cloth while it was prepared. The runaway tried hard not to look too hungry when the scrambled eggs on toast was set before her. There was even a small piece of fresh parsley perched in the middle of the bright yellow fluffy eggs. She did not want to waste time, and had fully intended to get the directions and hurry off, but her empty stomach had enticed her to accept the meal. The lady of the house was chatting away with her when there was a further knock on their front door.

    A car had pulled up on the gravel drive-way and the driver of the vehicle was quickly shown into the kitchen. Shirley was mortified. The priest, Father O'Rourke, from St. Josephs walked

Someone to Watch Over Me

in with a scowl on his rounded face. She started to run for the back door but he was quick, in spite of his rotund body, and he grabbed her and held her firmly until she calmed down. Without a word she was pushed and pulled out of the house and into the car and swiftly transported back to the orphanage.

The frightened girl was very upset in the car, fearing the punishment that lay ahead, but the priest reassured her that all would be forgiven. He explained that the people in the house had realised that she must have run away. The man of the house had telephoned to see if they had lost anyone from St. Josephs. Everyone was very embarrassed, but would be glad that Shirley was safe.

"Here you are little one. Thank the Lord that you are alright. I was out of my mind with worry that something awful must have happened to you. What a silly girl you were to run away. What do you think people will think? And after all that we do for you. How ungrateful. Come on then, let's get you settled into bed. Make sure that you don't wake the others, won't you."

Sister Gertrude seemed to be handling everything very well and Shirley relaxed a little as Sister said goodnight to Father O'Rourke. The minute he was out the door, long fingers with sharp nails bit into her arm and nasty words were spoken into her ear.

"I will make sure that you will never, ever, ever pull a stunt like that again. In the name of God you will never forget this Shirley Gilfillan. You are an evil little ungrateful wretch and you are going to be very, very sorry for what you have done this day, when I have finished with you."

The terrified child could feel the nun shaking with rage as she threatened her, her face right in Shirley's, spitting out her words which were soaked in venom.

"I'm sorry Sister. I didn't mean any harm. I just wanted to find the nice couple who took me to their lovely home......"

The nun cut her off with a sharp slap across her face and an angry snort like a fierce bull, pulling her roughly towards the stairs.

"Where are you taking me? You told Father O'Rourke that you were putting me to bed....."

"That's exactly what I am doing....afraid of the dark are you Shirley? And scared of small spaces are you Shirley? Scared of being alone are you Shirley? I found out just the right punishment for you by listening to your friends."

The nasty nun was dragging and pulling the child up the stairs all the time she was spitting out her nasty threats. At one stage she had grabbed Shirley's hair and had dragged her by that as well as her arm, her nails biting into flesh.

She half dragged and half pushed the terrified child up into the darkness and along a passageway into a tiny room with only a small bed and a hand basin. Shirley looked around frantically and could see a room adjacent to it with a desk in it. She had not seen this part of the building before.

The woman with evil on her mind, pushed the child into the tiny room. She closed and locked the door into the adjoining office. It was cold in the room. The nun turned off the light and then reached up to the lightbulb, unscrewed it and placed it in her pocket. She slammed the door shut, turned the key in the lock and the terrified child heard her walk away. The little bit of light that had shone from the staircase was now shut out and Shirley could see nothing. She stumbled to the bed and kicked something as she fell onto the small cot. She screamed. She pulled herself together and kicked it again. It must be a chamber pot. At least she had that should she need to use it.

Feeling abandoned, rejected and despised, she felt for a blanket and discovered that there wasn't one. There was a pillow without a pillowcase, a sheet on the mattress and a thin cotton bedspread. She climbed under the covering, fully clothed to keep warm, and tried to stop shivering. Shirley tried to pretend she

Someone to Watch Over Me

was in the lovely bed with the lace cover at Mr. and Mrs. Wilson's place. She tried to make out that she was warm. She tried to forget that the space was small and very dark and that she was locked in and all alone.

Chapter Eighteen

'Calm me O Lord, as You stilled the storm,
Still me, O Lord, keep me from harm,
Let all the tumult within me cease,
Enfold me, Lord, in Your peace.'
Celtic Traditional

It had been a particularly cold autumn night and Shirley was terribly unhappy. It was raining outside and the wind was howling. Each new sound frightened the lonely girl even more. She snuggled down under the thin bedcover, which was no thicker than a sheet. She had left even her shoes on, but even this did not help to keep her warm. She was freezing. She needed to use the chamber pot, but was too scared to get out of bed in the pitch blackness. She held on and curled herself up into a tight ball on the lumpy mattress.

Cold, lonely, and scared, she watched the light appear around the blind in the window. At first it was a dull grey. Gradually she was able to make out shapes in the room. There was a crucifix over the bed. There was a glass on the hand basin. She would not have to cup her hands for a drink, as they needed to in the dormitory. She could see the door clearly now. It was painted to match the pale greyish colour of the walls. There was a large brass door knob and underneath, a large key hole. She quickly jumped out of bed and looked through the key hole, but could see nothing. The key was still in it. She put her ear to the door to hear if anyone was coming. Silence.

Hurriedly, she pulled down her panties as she pulled the chamber pot out from under the bed. She looked under the bed first to see if anyone nasty was under it. All night she had imagined horrible creatures and grotesque people waiting there to do terrible things to her. She chastised herself, in the light of day, for all of the frightening thoughts that had raced through her mind in the darkness and loneliness of this little room.

It seemed like a whole day passed before someone came. Shirley quickly arranged herself in a lady-like sitting position on the bed and waited. *At last they will let me go back down to my friends,* she thought.

She was relieved.

The door to the rest of the world opened. Standing there like the grim reaper himself was Sister Gertrude. Shirley braced herself for a huge lecture, telling herself not to answer back but to say she was sorry and then it would be over, at last.

"Getting hungry yet are you? You horrid little wretch. I'm not done with you yet. Oh no I'm not. Try to pull a fast one on me would you? Try to run away from all of us here who have slaved our fingers to the bone taking such good care of you? What a hateful little throw-away piece of rubbish you are. No wonder nobody wants you and you've ended up here. Now we have to do what we can to make a decent person out of you. More work for us. Well, we'll obey our God-given calling and we'll make sure that you are no longer wicked. You'll be good if it kills me in the process."

"I'm sorry Sister, really I am. I didn't mean to cause any trouble. Please, I just want to go back down with my friends."

"Ha! You don't really think that is going to happen in a hurry do you? It will be a long time before you see any of them again."

With this terrifying threat, Sister Gertrude drew a belt from behind her back and started lashing out at the defenceless girl. The screaming child tried to fight off the belt with her hands, pleading for mercy. Her cries were ignored by her tall, spiteful, crazed jailer who was chanting all the time as she belted her.

"In the name of the Father," another lash across her arm "and the name of the Son," as the belt lashed her back, "and the name of the Holy Spirit" as it swung across her thigh.

Shirley lay on the bed sobbing and hurting all over. The nun was silent now and out of breath. She opened the door, staggering through the doorway and pulled it closed, locking it behind her.

It was night-time before Shirley heard someone outside the door again. She quickly jumped up and moved to the corner of the room, terrified that her tormentor had returned.

"Wh-wh-wh-who is it?" she stammered, in the dark room. The key turned in the lock and the door was opened.

A hand reached out to turn on the light, flicking the switch several times.

"What has happened to the light Shirley?"

It was Sister Cecilia.

"Why are you crouching over there? Whatever is the matter?'

The nun walked over to the distressed child and could see that she was terrified.

"You must be hungry. I have brought you up something to eat." She paused for a moment and then whispered "Are you alright?"

Shirley no longer trusted anyone. Not even Sister Cecilia.

"Y-y-y-yes Sister. I a-a-am alright. B-b-b-but very hungry. Th-th-thank you."

"I will empty your chamber pot child. Enjoy the food while I do."

She disappeared out of the door and down the hall.

Shirley quickly gulped down the stew that had a piece of bread sitting on top of it. She was pleased to see that Sister had included a glass of milk. She had not realised how hungry she was until she saw the food, or how lonely for a friend she was until she heard the gentle voice of Sister Cecilia.

Chapter Nineteen

'What worries you masters you.'   Haddon W. Robinson

The children downstairs were whispering. Somehow they had found out that their little friend was in trouble. It had been days since she had run away and someone had talked in the kitchen about a meal for the child 'in solitary.' Muriel was on kitchen duties and she overheard the sister say that it was for the girl who ran away, and that she was locked away until she learned her lesson. She also heard her say that the girl would only get one meal a day and no company, light or warmth.

The children were quieter than usual. Meal times were subdued. Bedtime was quiet. Even the little ones were worried about Shirley. She had been kind to them, always trying to cheer them up when they were missing their families. Sometimes the comfort came as a piece of stolen peel from the rubbish bin or red berries from the forbidden bush. If they forgot their jackets in the morning, no-one was allowed to go back inside except for meals, school, kitchen duties or the toilet, and they had to stay cold all day, and she would chase them around the yard to get them warm. It had become her passion, looking out for the little ones. She was now one of the big girls and it was one of her duties to take care of the small ones.

Her friends Muriel, Anna and Jacinta and their little cousin Bobby talked together anxiously.

"Shirley will be terrified. She hates being alone. Her uncle had to leave her alone a lot and she can't stand it."

Poor Jacinta shared her concerns and burst into tears.

"The room where they have her is tiny. She'll be real scared. And there is nothing in it for her to do. She'll go nuts."

Muriel was the oldest and had managed to find out about 'the cell.'

"She'll be starving with only one small meal a day."

Anna was the practical one and she noticed everything. She was also a straight talker who made every word count.

Bobby had been very thoughtful and he suddenly spoke up.

"Poor Shirley, she hates the dark. I hope she has a lamp at night."

He sucked on his two middle fingers, eyes large and sad for his friend.

After seven long, cold and lonely days and nights, the ten year old girl was let out of solitary confinement. She stood silently on the stairs, her menacing abuser towering over her. Shirley still wore the clothes she had run away in, but now she wore a different expression. The broken girl looked like a frightened kitten and jumped when her jailer spoke. The nun addressed all of the children who had been assembled to witness Shirley's return to the community.

"Children, I want you to look at this girl. She has been punished for her sins and we have now forgiven her. She is sorry for running away. Do not think of trying to run away yourselves or you too will receive the same punishment. Thank you, you can return outside until lunch time."

Sister Gertrude marched down the stairs with a nasty curl to her lips, which looked more like a sneer than a smile. Shirley crept down the stairs like a frightened little mouse, terrified of a cat pouncing at any moment.

Shirley was different. She did not join in with the activities as before her imprisonment. She stuttered if she spoke and spoke so quietly it was a strain to hear her words.

Someone to Watch Over Me

The young girl tried very hard to please everyone, especially the nuns. She sat with her back straight and her hands clasped in 'chapel' and did not whisper secretly to her friends, as before.

The children were quiet too, for a long time. Their little friend's change did not escape anyone's notice. Shirley's ill treatment had traumatised the whole orphanage. It was a long time before any other child attempted escape. The sisters had won again.

Someone to Watch Over Me

Chapter Twenty

'Hope begins in the dark, the stubborn hope that if you just show up and try to do the right thing, the dawn will come. You wait and watch and work; you don't give up.'   Anne Lamott

"The Lord Jesus is real, and He hasn't forgotten me."

Shirley was excited that her prayers seemed to be answered. Every night when she had gone to bed she had taken out something from under her pillow. It was the one possession that the nuns had given all the children for a Christmas present. It was a photo of the Holy painting of the Son of God with the bleeding heart. She had prayed to this photo which she treasured.

She longed to leave the orphanage. Sister Gertrude had continued to be nasty to her ever since she had run away. Shirley was very scared of her and tried to be submissively obedient, but she always seemed to be singled out and punished. Ridicule was the sister's favourite tool against her and she especially liked to poke fun at her blind eye. Shirley's eyes were a pretty bright blue and you had to look very closely to see that one was damaged. However, the nun would call her 'bung-eye' when she felt like it and taunt her not to lose the sight in her good eye or she would 'really be in the dark.'

This morning she had been called into the office and Sister Gertrude had advised her that she would be going to live in the country to help an old couple, It was near the Flinders Ranges and she was a very lucky girl indeed. She was informed that if she did what she was told and worked hard, she would be able to stay there indefinitely. Shirley looked down, choosing not to look at the nun who continued to taunt her. If she had, she would have been confused to see the woman looking very pleased with herself. The child whispered "thank you" and hurried off to find her friends.

It would be sad to say 'goodbye' to the three girls who had become her special friends. She dreaded the thought of farewelling little Bobby too. She knew that he would be very upset to see his friend and ally leave 'the home' and move on with her life. Shirley knew, however, that at ten years of age she had to make the most of whatever opportunity came her way. She had given up all hope that any of her real family would come for her.

"Did you know that Ella went to a place that sounded like the one that you are going to? She hated it. She came back very upset. Why don't you see if she'll tell you what it was like?"

Anna was always the realist in the group. She had learned at an early age to question everyone and everything. Trust was not something she did.

Shirley eagerly sought out Ella in the yard after breakfast. She quickly established that Ella had indeed gone to the same place, to a house in Carrieton where a Mr. and Mrs. McArdle lived.

"Actually, it was not their place, but they were caretakers for the owner, and as they were elderly, they needed help around the house."

Other than that, Ella would say nothing. She did, however, whisper to Shirley to be very wary and to watch out for the old man. She said to never be alone with him, he was nasty and he was 'a dirty old man.'

Shirley shrugged off the dark cloud that had gathered around her since talking with Anna and then Ella, and decided to look at what lay ahead as an adventure and a holiday of sorts.

Within days she was hugging and kissing her friends goodbye. She felt churned up and her feelings were all mixed together into a real mess. *A bit like the children's clothes in the clean laundry basket*, she thought to herself.

One second she felt excited and nervous and then she felt terribly sad and guilty as she looked at the dearly loved faces of her envious, yet concerned friends.

Suddenly she was brought back to reality as she felt a rough push in the back. It was Mr. McArdle, who had driven down to Adelaide to collect her.

"Come on girl. I don't have all day. I hope you're not always so slow to get started. The car's over there. Move yourself."

Shirley thought that the old car looked like it had travelled quite a few miles. She thought Mr. McArdle looked like he had too. She and her little case were deposited in the back seat and the car was soon moving off towards the gates. This time she was exiting legally. She looked over her shoulder as they drove off, savouring her last look at her best friends. They were waving sadly. She looked at the place they secretly called 'The house of horrors' and hoped that she would never see it again. A tear rolled down her cheek as she saw Jacinta and Bobby in tears.

Sister had told her that they would be driving to Rosewater to Mr. McArdle's niece's place and would stay there overnight. He wanted to get some business done, and then they would take off early next morning for Carrieton.

"What's it like where you live?" asked the nervous child.

"It's a long trip to Carrieton, so I want to get away at sun-up. Don't keep me waiting" he barked.

Other than that, he did not speak with her all of the way to his niece's house.

What an old grump, thought the ten year old. She decided to give up any further attempts at conversation until they reached their destination.

Just looking at the scenery as they drove past was enough for her anyway. The colourful gardens were such a treat after the drabness of St. Joseph's. She realised how starved she was for colour and drank it in as they drove up the streets and past houses, cars, shops and people. Shirley was delighted to see people. Normal people. They were chatting in the street, tidying their gardens, or walking along as if they did not have a care in the world. Some of them were smiling and holding the hands of a child or two, or walking a dog. There were children playing cricket in the street and calling and laughing out loud. Some couples were out pushing a pram and chatting to each other as they strolled along. Sights and sounds that were unfamiliar yet yearned for in Shirley's short and troubled life. Images of normality and joy and love. Images that she would capture in her mind forever and treasure like precious family photographs.

The young girl allowed her thoughts to travel on ahead to Carrieton. Would she make some friends there? Would the people like her? Would she get to go shopping and to church and to play in the street with other children? Would there be fancy teas and grand people visiting? Maybe someone would love her and she could become part of a family. This could be a new beginning for her. She sat up in her seat and fixed her hair as best she could, without seeing in a mirror, or using a brush or comb. Looking down at her drab clothes, badly matched and worn, she hoped that country folk would not be too critical of her appearance, but make allowances for a child who was dressed from 'the poor box.'

Chapter Twenty One

'Hope is the thing with feathers that perches in the soul.' Emily Dickinson

The old car turned into a gravel driveway, lined with bright red geraniums. It came to a halt and the old man pulled on the hand brake. Shirley did not move. He had not spoken for miles and she was a little scared of him because of the silence between them.

The tension was broken by the appearance of a young woman wearing a red checked and cross-stitched apron, holding a tea-towel in her hands. She wore a cheery smile as well and warmly greeted her uncle with a kiss to his cheek.

"About time you got here. I was about to send out a search party. Whatever took you so long? I have been getting very impatient, thinking you may have decided not to come this way after all. Aren't you going to introduce me to this adorable little curly-top in your back-set? She looks like a little princess sitting there so grandly." Shirley was blushing like the geraniums and couldn't help smiling at the warmth of her chauffeur's young niece.

"Her name is Shirley. Like the little kid in the pictures. The nun says that she is quite good in the kitchen, so let's hope she lives up to her reputation. Poor old Mrs. McArdle is getting a bit past it with her aches and pains, you know."

He was mumbling under his breath as he left the young girl to get out of the car with her case.

Someone to Watch Over Me

"Shirley is it? I love the name Shirley. I used to have a dolly that I called Shirley just because I loved the name so much. Well, young Shirley, I can see that my uncle has forgotten his manners. He never was any good with words. My name is Nell and I am very happy for you to call me that. I am newly married and my husband is called Will. He will be along in a tick. He and Uncle are going to do a bit of business while you and I get to know each other. Would you like to see your room? We can take your case there."

Nell reached down and took it out of the hands of the obviously shy girl.

They walked through the tidy garden to the front door and Shirley was impressed with the polished veranda. She thought to herself how even all the sisters put together would not be able to find a dull spot. The front door was ajar and an arrogant-looking ginger cat eyed her off with suspicion. Shirley quickly squatted to stroke the cat, taken with its glorious markings. It closed its eyes, purring and made friends with her immediately.

"Well, I never," said Nell.

"Megs never takes to anyone that fast. You must have a special way with cats. You like them do you?"

"M-m-my grandmother had a cat and I always l-l-l-loved to nurse her and s-s-stroke her. She s-s-s-slept on my bed when I v-visited."

The child was relieved to find something to talk about.

"See, I knew it. You do have a special knack with cats. Megs does not make new friends easily."

Nell was leading the child through the house to the end of the passageway where a white-painted door stood shut and waiting.

"Here we are Shirley. This room is for our special visitors. We do not let just anyone stay here. Come along now and tell me if you like it.'"

Nell was anxious to see Shirley relax a little as she could tell that she was extremely nervous, especially around her Uncle.

Someone to Watch Over Me

Nell opened the door and Shirley was bathed in the welcoming feeling of the room.

There was a pretty, patterned patchwork quilt on the bed and the biggest doll that she had ever seen sitting on it, with her lacy, knitted skirt spread out all around her. There was a shelf along the wall and on it were many different sized books. Some were very thin, some small, and some were huge. The covers were various colours and Shirley's fingers itched to open them and see if there were pictures inside. Because reading was such a struggle for her, she was drawn to books with pictures. There was a painted dressing table with a little skirt of pretty fabric covering the legs. Hooks hung on another wall with a jaunty hat perching on one and an old leather school bag hanging from another.

The friendly hostess noticed Shirley's eyes darting back to a covered basket sitting alongside the dressing table.

"That's my sewing basket. Would you like to lift the lid and see what is inside? It is full of all sorts of treasures. My mother gave it to me because she would dearly love me to sew, but I am afraid that I am a failure. I never had the patience to learn and I am afraid to say that I can't even sew on a button."

Shirley's eyes opened wide with her eyebrows expressing surprise."

"I-I-I thought that you must h-h-have made the beautiful b-b-bedspread."

As soon as she had spoken she quickly regretted her words and her hands went to her mouth.

"I'm s-s-sorry, I didn't m-m-mean anything, really I d-d-didn't."

She looked like she was about to cry and Nell felt alarmed.

"You didn't say anything wrong, Rosebud. I just wish I had taken notice when my mother tried to teach me. If only I could darn, or sew on a button, I wouldn't feel so bad. My clever Mum made the bedspread and all of the other nice things you can see around the house."

Someone to Watch Over Me

"I-I-I c-c-could teach you."

Shirley had blurted it out before she knew it.

Nell's whole body responded with pleasure as she grabbed up her sewing basket and flopped on to the bouncy bed.

"Come on then, let's get started right away. Uncle can fend for himself and you and I will have a sewing lesson. Who taught you then? Was it your Gran or did you learn it at St. Jo's?"

After a couple of hours they were good friends and laughed together as Nell exaggerated her clumsiness with threading the needle and kept losing the thread from the eye of the needle as she attempted to sew a few running stitches and then attempted to darn a sock.

The old man and Will had been talking out on the veranda and drinking beer. Eventually Will wandered in to meet their little visitor. He was lots of fun and Shirley found herself sitting nursing Megs and laughing as Will teased her and told her stories of his work at the general store.

"Where's my tucker, wife?" he asked jovially.

"What are we having? Don't tell me it's tripe again. I couldn't stand it. Do you know what tripe is girlie? It comes from the lining of the cow's stomach. It's a bit like eating the sole of an old shoe. Taste's just about as good too."

Shirley was smiling and she felt happy for the first time in a long time. She looked around the room taking in the pretty things everywhere. Nellie seemed to know just what was needed to cheer up a corner and the whole house seemed happy. Even the toilet out the back had magazines in a special holder and a pretty basket with artificial flowers in it and cut up newspaper for toilet paper.

She cheered me up just the same, thought the sensitive and grateful girl.

The smile on her face widened as she looked at her new friends, Nell and Will with affection. They were so comfortable with each other and were madly in love.

Suddenly her mood changed. Out of the corner of her eye she saw the old man staring at her. He still had not spoken one word to her, but he was looking at her in a most peculiar way. A shudder went through her and she quickly looked away.

"Alright then, husband, I'll tell you what is for tea. It's my famous specialty. It's salmon patties. So what do you think about that?"

Nell looked adoringly at her husband for his approval.

"And is our little cook going to show you how to make them properly?" he teased, with a wink.

"What a good idea that would be Will. She has already spent the whole afternoon teaching me to sew, so we might as well get her to teach me to cook as well."

Nell picked up on Will's efforts to include Shirley in the conversation and did not miss his wink across the kitchen table.

"But I have n-n-never made s-s-salmon p-p-patties," said Shirley, a little worried.

"What. Do you mean that I am going to get to teach you something for a change Rosebud? That would only be fair, heh?"

Shirley jumped up from her chair as Nell did and before anyone could say 'Jack Robinson' they were busying themselves with potatoes and saucepans, an onion and carrots and peas, an egg, some flour and butter. Shirley opened the can of salmon and expertly drained the juice into a glass.

"Will likes to drink the juice, so I'm glad you saved it. Well done."

Shirley was glowing with the praise and wanted more of it. She loved working alongside Nell and couldn't believe how much fun it could be cooking without someone watching, ready to pounce on you with words of scorn should you make a mistake.

Dinner was served with lemon wedges from their tree out the back and the food looked pretty with the different colours on the plates. Will watched Shirley around Nell and could tell that the child liked her new friend and had thoroughly enjoyed herself working alongside her. He excused himself and disappeared for a short time. When he returned he had something behind his back that he teased the young girl with for a moment.

"No lassie, it is not something that bites. Not most of the time anyway. Here, take a look and tell me if you would like it."

"It is a l-l-lovely photo, W-W-Will. D-D-Do you mean it? Can I r-r-really have it to k-k-keep?"

It was a photograph of Nell, taken on their honeymoon. It was taken out in the country and she was laughing with her hair blowing in the breeze. She looked radiant. Shirley loved it.

"It's yours curly-top. You can keep it as a reminder of your stay with Will and Nell. Then you won't forget us too quickly."

The look on Shirley's face cut to his heart. She looked shocked at his even entertaining the idea that she would ever forget her time with them. He so wished that they could afford to pay the Catholics to have her stay with them and help Nell. He hoped that they would have a baby on the way before long and Nell would have loved the company and the help. He knew that Shirley would be very sad to leave in the morning. Especially with Nell's grumble bum Uncle. He hoped that she would survive those two horrid people and that there would be some children in the township of Carrieton willing to be her friends.

Carrieton was a small town, located about 100 kilometres east of Pt. Augusta. It was on the southern edge of the Flinders Ranges and in the middle of nowhere. Temperatures could sour in Summer and the nights in Winter could be very cold.

Hope they don't work the girlie too hard, thought Will, knowing what those two oldies were like. *If either of them smiled, their faces would crack. Fair dinkum.*

Mr. McArdle pushed his chair back from the table with a loud scrape.

"I'm off." He spoke gruffly as he headed for his bed.

"I'll knock on your door to wake you. Make sure you don't keep me waiting."

With that he was gone. Shirley helped with the clearing of the table and the dishes and said her fond 'goodnights' to her new friends. Before long she was tucked into her bed with the colourful quilt and was cherishing thoughts of the lovely time spent with Will and Nell. When she thought of how Will had teased her and called her 'Curly-top' she smiled to herself and snuggled down further under the cosy covers.

The whole household seemed to be asleep very quickly and all that could be heard was the ticking of the chiming clock on the mantel in the sitting room. Shirley loved lying there listening to it. It triggered memories of her grandmother's house. It reminded her of her father with the prickly moustache, standing by the fireplace winding the mantle clock with the Westminster chimes. The lonely girl wrapped her arms around herself as the memories brought pain. She tried to forget, rocking herself to sleep as she struggled to wipe out the mental picture of 'family'. Finally she drifted off.

Someone to Watch Over Me

Chapter Twenty Two

'In the end we will remember not the words of our enemies, but the silence of our friends.' Martin Luther King Jr.

All the way to Carrieton she could not look at him. He had placed her in the front seat this time and she stayed as close to the door as she could. She could sense him though and the feeling of threat wrapped itself around her shoulders like a dark cape.

Saying goodbye to Nell and Will was hard. She had grown so fond of them very quickly. Their kindness and warmth was a foreign experience in her harsh and cold world. The 'goodbye' was even more painful because they represented protection and safety to the vulnerable child. She was being driven off into the unknown by a threatening stranger. He was an unfriendly guardian who had given nothing to her at this stage to reassure her or show that he cared one spot about her feelings.

Silence hung between them for miles until he finally spoke, sending chills up and down her spine. "You will do exactly what I ask when we get to Carrieton. You will speak to no-one, only Mrs. McArdle and myself. We have paid for you and we own you. No-one cares about you and no-one will come to rescue you. Do you understand?" He was looking at her.

"Look at me when I speak to you." The words were a snarl. She slowly turned her head in his direction and their eyes held. His were dark and menacing and hers scared but defiant.

She looked away from him at the passing scenery. Her heart was pounding in her chest. She made herself concentrate on the view through the window. The distant hills were beautiful. They were all sorts of purples and mauves and the sky was an amazing cobalt blue. Vivid colour, with large white fluffy clouds clinging to the lavender horizon. Her Uncle Charlie could paint and he had pointed out different colours to her, teaching her their names. She loved gum trees and they were passing some giants with spectacular markings on their pale trunks. Unique patterns as if some eccentric artist had come with his variegated palette and chosen gums at random to mark with purples, browns, greys and reds. The bark hung in large pieces here and there as the trees shed their skin like huge snakes. She especially loved the colours of the long, tapered leaves that hung in clumps, like fingers, displaying many different shades of grey, green and blue.

"Do you hear me?" This time the words were slow and deliberate and sneering.

She would not answer him. But she nodded slightly, once.

He grabbed at her across the space between them.

"I will do whatever I want with you and you will co-operate. There is no-one to help you. Get it?"

He was squeezing her arm until she knew it would be bruised. Brute force with one arm while he drove the car along the purple ribbon of road with the other.

This is not happening to me. Some other little girl is being frightened by this ugly, horrible old man, she thought.

She had started to pretend in this way while she was locked in solitary confinement in 'the prison room.' She considered jumping out of the car. She inched her hand towards the door handle.

Quick little one. Save yourself and jump. This was happening to another young girl, she thought. Her hand was on the handle.

"No use thinking of jumping out of the car. There's no-one on the road today. No-one will come along and save you. Only the eagles waiting until you die and then they will pluck out your eyes and tear the flesh from your bones."

Someone to Watch Over Me

He started to laugh. It was an evil laugh. Mean and cruel. Like a demon from hell that the nuns talked about.

She was not giving up. When they got to the house he couldn't watch her all of the time. Maybe Mrs. McArdle would help her and let her use the telephone. She might be able to pretend that she forgot to tell Nell something and be able to make a call and blurt out to them to come and save her. They would, she knew they would. They liked her and would remember her and be very upset that she was in such desperate circumstances.

She thought of the little girl who was not her but someone else and she felt sorry for her. Shirley was alright, everything was alright. Mr. McArdle was a nice man and he was taking her to a lovely house in the country where she would help the old couple with a few chores, in exchange for her keep. It was a fresh start for her and she was going to love Carrieton.

She closed her eyes and tried to believe all that was true.

Deep, deep down, though, where the truth resided, she knew she was in great trouble. She knew that there was no escape. She quickly closed the door on those thoughts and told herself that she was quite safe and everything was a new adventure. She did feel sorry for the little girl, though, who was in terrible trouble and terrified of what might lay ahead down the road.

Chapter Twenty Three

'The godly can look forward to a reward, while the wicked can expect only judgement.' Proverbs 11:3

Each morning Shirley had to rise early to feed the chooks and collect the eggs. Whilst there in the yard she had to go to the front of the house to pump water and carry the bucket into the kitchen. There was no water on tap in the house and Carrieton was a hot and dry place where water was respected. She was careful not to spill a drop. Mrs. McArdle had screamed at her when she had a little mishap on the first morning.

Mr. McArdle had been waiting at the pump for her in his old checkered shirt, overalls and dusty leather boots. He looked like anyone's quaint old grandpa, but she knew differently. He glared at her and she tried to ignore him.

"Cat got your tongue?" He growled his words at her like a hungry dog.

"Good morning." She spoke as coolly as she dared and quickly filled the bucket from the pump. As she pumped he moved closer. The hairs stood up on the back of her neck and she glanced frantically towards the farm house, hoping to see Mrs. McArdle in the kitchen window.

"She won't be up for hours. Came down with the 'flu through the night."

He spoke menacingly, with no concern for his elderly wife's health. He grabbed at Shirley's top, tugging her towards him. The frightened girl pulled away and ran for her life, leaving the capsized bucket at the pump, with the precious water making a large puddle on the thirsty ground. She must hide somewhere. He was after her and she was unprotected. Where could she go? Not her bedroom. It was just a sleep out at the back of the house. There was only a curtain to pull across the opening and no doors to lock. She ran as fast as her little legs could carry her, to the house and then down the side and around the back. She tore past the chook shed then stopped to look over her shoulder to see if she was being chased.

Shirley was breathing heavily from both fear and exertion. She heard him, cursing and grunting before she saw him. She was crouching behind the corrugated iron sheets which formed the walls of the chook shed. She was out of sight but she knew that he could guess where she was. She crept further away from where she had last seen him and tried not to breath but crouch silently, curled into a ball of fear and dread.

"Gotcha!"

He sprang from the other end and grabbed her with both hands, forcing her up and onto her feet. Shirley screamed and fought him, struggling to get away. It was useless. He was tall and strong and overpowered her.

"Please don't. Let me go. Leave me alone. Help me. Someone help me."

She screamed again, stirring up the hens this time and causing panic in the chook house.

There was no-one. She was defenceless. Mrs. McArdle didn't seem interested in helping her at other times, and now that she was ill there was no hope that she would intervene.

Her eyes were wide with fear and her hands shook. She knew what was going to happen and at the thought she vomited.

"You filthy pig. You threw up on me. Now I stink as bad as you."

He grabbed his handkerchief from his pocket and started wiping himself down. Shirley saw her chance and darted for the house. She ran to the back door, slamming the screen door behind her and looked around frantically seeking a hiding place. She ran past her bedroom with the pull curtain for a door, through the small kitchen and into Mrs. McArdle's room. The old lady woke with a start at her unexpected visitor and Shirley asked between gulps of breath if she could bring her anything.

"You stink, girl. A cup of tea in a minute. First of all get me the chamber pot from under the bed."

She saw him watching through the window and then shrug his shoulders and walk off into the vegetable garden. The child had escaped……. this time.

Chapter Twenty Four

"As for me, I am poor and needy; please hurry to my aid, O God. You are my helper and my saviour. O Lord do not delay." Psalm 70:5

Shirley worked very hard at her chores. There was no entertainment to distract her and nowhere to go. The isolated house was miles from the town. She thought a lot about running away, but could see the futility of doing so. She knew that the old man would chase her in his car and any of the townspeople would hold her until he came and picked her up. Just like the time when she tried to escape from the orphanage. She thought of running to the open road, but had no confidence that strangers would believe her and help her. She had to work out a plan and be brave. Escape was going to be a challenge. It occupied her every thought and at night she lay on her bed dreaming up schemes that didn't stand up to her daylight scrutiny.

She washed by hand and ironed with the old coal-filled box iron, cooked, carted water and washed dishes. The hours were long. She worked from dawn until dusk every day with no time off. Her only outings were the occasional trip into town to help with the shopping and the mandatory trip to the pretty little church on the hill each Sunday morning. St. Raphael's church sat there looking impressive on the fringe of the small town. The local Catholics came religiously in their cars or horse drawn carts each Sunday morning, rain or shine.

Someone to Watch Over Me

Shirley liked going to the church because it gave her the opportunity to see other people, and especially other children. She loved the music and would join in the singing. The spectacle of the priest in his pristine robes pleased her and stirred her memories of earlier experiences back at the orphanage. However, there was a price to pay each Saturday night in preparation for church next morning.

"The bucket of water is near the car. I've left some old rags there too. See that you make it shine ready for church."

He did not look at Shirley. He continued to finish his dinner while he waved her out of the house.

The girl pulled her tired body out of the chair and dragged herself out to the shed. It was a short walk from the house and she was always afraid that one of the scary rats that she saw scuttling around the yard at twilight might appear. She knew that they were there, but did not want to see them. It was still light as it was summer and the sun had not gone to rest as yet. She was ready for bed. It may have been Saturday, but she had risen at 5:30am to do her chores and had been working all day. This was her last responsibility for the day, but it was the most dreaded chore of all.

He would sneak out on Saturday night to the shed and torment her, while she was trying to clean the buckboard. First he would talk his "stupid talk" about her being his little wife and taking good care of all of his needs. Then he would mumble about how bad it was having babies and that she must not get pregnant. He sometimes said that having babies was worse than having your leg chopped off. She had no idea what he meant by all of that, but was terrified of having babies and prayed to the Lord, desperately, that she would not get pregnant. Shirley did not know exactly what made a girl get pregnant, but she had a few ideas.

She hoped that he would get busy and not come to the shed tonight. He still had his dessert to eat. It was rhubarb and custard. They had a little vegetable plot down near the chook shed and he had picked some rhubarb and told her to cook it for tea. The custard was her idea. Seeing there was plenty of milk in the ice chest, she decided to make a nice, thick, egg custard. It ended up with a few lumps, but overall it was not bad and she felt proud of her efforts, made on the ancient wood stove.

She knew that he would eat his sweets and then have his usual sweet cup of tea before coming out to the shed. Her plan was to work very quickly, and not too fussily, to enable her to get back into the house before he appeared She washed and rubbed and wiped up the suds as fast as her arms would go. She was exhausted but as she had heard Mrs. McArdle say many times "where there's a will there's a way." The old lady did not talk very much, and was mean and prickly, but Shirley was used to mean and prickly women so she tried to ignore her. She worked furiously and was almost finished, when she heard footsteps coming into the shed. Her heart sank and she felt a great disappointment swamp her like heavy, icy rain.

Not tonight. Please, not tonight. I can't stand it. Not again.

Her words were not spoken out loud, but screamed inside her head. She was terrified of the old man, and the nasty things that he threatened to do to her if she disobeyed him, or told their secret.

"Take off your clothes Shirley and get into the car with me."

With her head hung low and a look of unbearable shame on her face, the slave obeyed her master.

She wanted to run, but what was the use. He had caught up with her every time. She knew by now that Mrs. McArdle would not rescue her. She had suspicions that she knew, but that she chose to turn her back on the monstrous abuse of the little girls that were sent out from St. Joseph's to work for them. Shirley thought of pretty little Ella, who had come here before her. She had bouncing blond curls and a sunny personality. When she had returned from this hellish place, she had not spoken to anyone for a long time, and only picked at her food for weeks. Finally Shirley knew why.

She let her mind drift off to a nicer place, pretending that the nasty things were happening to another little girl. She was sitting in a very smart car with the nice young couple who bought her the green velvet dress with the stunning cape. She was wearing it now and they were all going on a picnic together. They were headed for a nice park and the birds were singing and the sun was shining. It was a perfect day and the sky was a lovely cobalt blue. There were swings in the park and she couldn't wait to swing back and forth way up into that pretty sky with the fluffy white clouds. She knew it would be marvellous fun and would feel like she had wings, just like the birds way up above.

That would be a good escape plan. If only she had wings and could fly somewhere safe. Any place other than this farm house with only a curtain for a bedroom wall, and her bed in a draughty sleep out and this unmentionable animal.

Chapter Twenty Five

"You gain strength, courage and confidence by every experience in which you really stop to look fear in the face. You are able to say to yourself "I lived through this horror. I can take the next thing that comes along." Eleanor Roosevelt

Old Mrs. McArdle was gravely ill. She had been on her bed for days and had hardly eaten. Her coughing had become worse and more frequent. Finally her husband had taken notice and packed her into the back seat of the dark green 1918 Buick and driven her to see the doctor in Orroroo. He had been gone a long time, and returned without her.

"W-w-where is she?" asked Shirley, tentatively.

"Hospital." He spoke disinterestedly.

"What's w-w-w-wrong with her?" The child was concerned that the woman would not return.

"Pneumonia. She'll get over it. She always does. Now... (he rubbed his hands together enthusiastically). "What's for tea?"

He started looking around the kitchen as if he expected a three course dinner to be prepared and ready.

"Where's my grub? You lazy good for nothin'. What have you been doing all afternoon? You'll get a taste of my belt if you don't get something on the table soon."

Shirley knew she had better think of something that would cook quickly and grabbed some eggs from the bowl on the cupboard and some bacon from behind the curtain in the pantry. She stoked up the fire in the wood stove and scraped out some dripping from the tin can on the sink into the frypan. It was sizzling before long and she put three pieces of bacon into the frypan, somewhat relieved when the delicious aromas wafted around the kitchen. She knew that he would know his meal would be ready in a couple of minutes and she was safe from one of his beatings.

She quickly laid the table and placed his usual linen serviette on his bread and butter plate. Butter was scraped onto a saucer and home-made tomato sauce in its glass bottle was placed alongside the plate with two slices of bread. She quickly checked that everything was how he liked it and realised that the eggs needed to go into the frypan and a drink needed to be poured for him. She had squeezed some lemons from the tree in the yard earlier and made up a lemon cordial with a stack of sugar. She knew that he liked this and it may sweeten up his black mood.

Within minutes she served up his eggs on the fried bread that he liked, dipped into milk before frying. The bacon was crispy and nicely browned and still piping hot when he came to the table.

He ate in silence, not even noticing that she had nothing in front of her to eat. Shirley had decided to fry an egg for herself once he had left the room. She filled the kettle from the jug of water on the sink and put some tea leaves in the teapot. The hand-knitted tea cosy was placed on the table, waiting for the teapot. She nervously checked to see if everything was the way he insisted it should be, then relaxed a little when she decided that she had followed the rules well.

When he finished his hot meal he asked for some apricot jam for his bread and she quickly moved to the pantry, sliding across the curtain and picking up the small bowl of jam, she carried it to the table. He spread butter on his bread and then jam as she busied herself making the pot of tea and putting the tea cosy on the teapot. She had placed a bowl of sugar on the table for his tea

Someone to Watch Over Me

and now took a deep breath recognising that all had gone well and he would retire to his room shortly.

He did just that and Shirley sat down in her chair with shoulders slumped, sighing deeply with relief. Feeling hungry she fried herself an egg and fried bread and ate it with the sweet taste of freedom from his tyrannical company. She could hear him snoring in his room and felt grateful that he would not bother her tonight with his dirty games.

After clearing up the kitchen she fell exhausted into bed and was soon asleep herself.

She woke with a start as someone lay down next to her. The birds were chirping their dawn song and she could see that the sun had woken up and was bringing everything to life. She moved away from him as he pulled the covers from the bed and grabbed at her.

"L-l-leave me alone. Go b-b-back to your own b-bed." She yelled at him, kicking and hitting out as he pulled at her nightie.

They fought and yelled at each other as he wrestled to overpower the eleven year old.

She screamed as he molested her.

"No. No. No." She yelled.

He attempted to rape her and she was sobbing now and still fighting him.

"What are you doing?!! Stop that. Leave her alone. She's only a child. You filthy pig."

The wicked old man's nephew had heard the screams and yelling and had raced around the side of the house to the back door. He could hardly believe his eyes when he saw his Uncle attempting to rape the child. The old man was found out. He had no defence. He turned on Shirley and started hitting her.

"You little hussy. Temptress! Vixen!"

As he went to hit her again his nephew grabbed his arm and pulled it back behind him, preventing him from hurting the child any more. He half sat on top of his uncle, yelling at him to calm down.

Shirley saw her chance to get away from the horrible scene and rolled off the bed, falling onto the floor, grabbing her clothes, then running through the curtain and into the kitchen. She was shaking all over with the shock of the whole awful scene and was shamed that the young man had seen what was being done to her. Finally the tears came, choking her as she broke down, hysterically crying and screaming until she collapsed onto the floor in front of the sink.

The young man came running into the kitchen, wanting to console her, but not knowing how to do so, recognising that the child was in a dreadful state. He raced back into the bedroom yelling at his now subdued uncle for the girl's name and grabbing the bedspread at the same time.

"Shirley," he spat out reluctantly.

The young man went back into the kitchen and tried to calm the girl by speaking gently and using her name, while he wrapped the bedspread around her.

"Shirley. Shirley. I am so sorry. I am so ashamed of my uncle. You poor girl. What can I do. I want to help but I don't know how. What if I telephone my sister, Nell? Nellie always knows what to do."

Shirley stopped screaming at the mention of Nell's name. He was Nell's brother. He was going to ring her. She would help her. It was going to end. All this torment was going to end. A tiny seed of hope started to grow in her heart. She would be rescued. Her prayers to Jesus were being answered. At last she would get away from this horrible place where dark things happened.

"W-w-why are y-y-you here?" she asked her rescuer.

"I had to go into Orroroo and pick up some supplies for the farm. It's about twenty miles from here. I heard about my aunt and was going to ask my uncle if he would like to come for the run and have a yarn on the way. I had to pass through Carrieton.

I'm so glad that I was here to help you. I'm going to ring Nell now."

Before long he was talking in hushed tones to his sister and trying to calm her down as she reacted as he expected to the awful news.

"Get that brute on the phone Jim. I'm going to scare the hell out of him."

Jim put the phone down and went back into the bedroom to fetch the disgraced monster who he once thought of as a fond uncle. He was subdued and staring into space, fearing the worst that would happen to him now.

"Nell wants to talk with you. Don't try to get out of this. You need to face the music. If you don't talk with her my next job is to ring the police."

The beaten old man dragged himself off the bed and into the kitchen where the telephone was on the wall. He knew that others could be listening in and the word would be all over the country like wildfire about his disgrace.

"Yeah. What do you want?"

"What I want from you is for you to go nowhere near that child ever again. I want you to realise that I could get in touch with the police and you could end up in deep trouble for your disgusting carryings on. How dare you. You make me sick. How could you?! You unspeakable brute. I never ever want to see you again. You dirty, disgusting, creepy piece of rubbish."

"What are you gunna do?" he asked with a trembling voice.

"I am going to get in touch with Will. As soon as he knocks off we are heading to Carrieton to pick up Shirley and bring her back to our place. Meanwhile I am going to phone St. Joseph's and once I have finished with them I am sure they will send a Social Worker to pick up this poor child and take her back to the home. You will NEVER get another child from there or anywhere else to abuse and use and make a slave of. You will leave the farm now and not come back until we have collected Shirley. Get out!!! Just go!!! If we see your face around the place when we get there I am going straight to the police. Now give the telephone back to Jim."

"Jim, are you there?"

"Yes I am Nell. I feel like being sick. What a b...........b........"

"I know Jimmy. I have a few choice names for the sod too. Let's concentrate on this child and doing all we can to fix this mess and help her to get over it. I shudder to think that this has been going on for all the months that she has been there.

"Can you make sure that the old creep gets off the property straight away? Are you able to hang around for a little while until Shirley is feeling a bit better? Maybe get her a drink and something to eat and settle her down a bit until we can get there?"

"Yes I can do that. Should I get in touch with the local priest? I'll ask Shirley if she'd like that."

"He's n-n-never spoken to m-m-me," stammered Shirley.

"Hasn't he come to visit and check on you love?"

Shirley sadly shook her head to say, "no."

Jim decided to forget involving him then, muttering his disapproval of this further neglect and abuse of a young girl, all alone in a strange place where she knew no-one.

"I am so sorry that we didn't check on you either, love. You must have felt completely abandoned. What sort of a crappy family are we?"

He was cross with himself, thinking what a happier time this child would have had in the country if someone had taken notice and looked out for her. He said "goodbye" to Nell and put on the kettle to make himself and his new little friend a cup of tea, with lots of sugar.

He told the dejected man to clear out and not come back until later that night. He met no opposition. Jim stayed as long as he could before he had to head off for Orrorro and the supplies that were needed for his father's farm, where he worked as a farm hand. He had telephoned earlier to put his parents in the picture and found that they had already heard on the "grapevine."

Mrs. Tilley had been listening in to his call with Nell and had been very quick to spread the dreadful news.

Ted McArdle drove into town, heading for the pub. He needed a drink or two. He couldn't see that he had done anything so awful. After all, the kid wasn't wanted by anyone. She was a reject. He had bought her from the orphanage and they didn't seem too worried about her. He was angry at the way he had been spoken to and treated. Even told to get off the farm. He was only having a bit of fun with the kid. She wasn't much good for anything else. She needed to pay for her keep, after all. He thought about how he'd like to pay back Nell and Jim and anyone else who wanted to point their self-righteous finger at him. He was a good church going, hard working man. Heaven help anyone in the town who judged him. He wouldn't stand for it. He would make sure that Nell and Will knew they were no longer welcome at the farm, or within "cooee" of him.

He sat at the bar drinking and then staggered to a table and chair in the corner. He downed several beers over as many hours and sulked into each schooner.

Suddenly the pub door flew open and Will was standing in front of him, hands on hips and his face red with anger.

"I knew I'd find you here. I dropped Nell off with Shirley so they can talk. I wanted to see you for myself. I could knock your block off. What sort of an animal are you?"

Ted didn't speak but he glared at Will with a look that could kill.

Will met his glare with his own and they stared at each other. The other people in the bar stared at both of them, expecting a fight to break out at any moment, even though one of the men was as old as the hills. Some of the men had heard the gossip but daren't say anything as was the culture of the day.

Someone to Watch Over Me

Will moved towards the perpetrator with fire in his eyes and shoved him in the chest.

"You are too old and decrepit for anyone worth his salt to take on. I'd make mince meat out of you in seconds. But I want you to hear what I have to say. Loud and clear. Nell and I disown you and will never have anything to do with you ever again. We wipe you out of our lives and turn our backs. You and I are finished in business and I will sort that out and let you know the outcome. Do not come near us or we will contact the police. You are an excuse for a human being. A worm. And the orphanage knows all about you and will spread the word to other child agencies. You are done for."

He nodded to the other men in the bar, tipped his hat and exited to his car.

There was deathly silence for several seconds and then everyone started talking about what had just happened. But no-one spoke to Ted McArdle.

Chapter Twenty Six

"I ask not for a lighter burden but for broader shoulders." A Jewish proverb

Nell and Shirley sat at the farm's kitchen table, sharing a cup of tea and their hearts. Shirley had cried a lot when Nell arrived at the property and the well had now dried up. Nell was overcome with compassion for this young girl who had endured so much in her very short life. Somehow Nell wanted to turn things around for her and promised herself that she would do her best. She had always believed that it was the tough things in life that broke us or made us strong. In fact, she liked the saying - "I'm yet to meet a strong person with an easy past."

She reached across the table and patted Shirley's hand.

"Life can be tough my dear - but so are you."

Shirley shrugged her shoulders to say that she wasn't sure about that.

The older woman continued to encourage her young friend until they heard Will drive up to the house and call out to them both. They both jumped up, glad of the shift of focus for a moment or two.

Will helped Shirley gather her few possessions into her case and then the three of them headed for the car, leaving the door open and gladly turning their backs on a place that neither of the three ever wanted to see again.

"Let's get some miles between this place and home as soon as we can. The old coot will come back before long. He's as drunk as a skunk right now so just as well he'll mainly be driving on a private dirt road."

Shirley hoped he'd have an accident and then asked God to forgive her, making a cross on her chest.

They bumped along the dry dusty road and Will tried to avoid the pot holes. He was travelling much faster than usual, and slowed down when he saw the gate that he needed to open and then close behind them. They were driving through another property in order to get back onto the main road out of Carrieton. Shirley jumped out of the car to help him and jumped when she saw a car approaching them.

"Oh no! "

Nell's hands went to her face when she saw that it was her Uncle's car. She quickly summoned the girl back into Will's car and Will jumped into the driver's seat and hit the accelerator. None of them wanted to speak any further with Ted McArdle and were horrified that he had come back so soon to the farm. Shirley's eyes were wide with fear as she saw him driving at a rate of knots towards the gate and then watched him swerve the steering wheel and accelerate towards them. The girls screamed and Will avoided a collision by steering off the road into the paddock. They kept going, and then Will brought the car back onto the dirt road again. The three finally took a breath and looked back over their shoulders. The old man had stopped the car just in time, without ramming the gate and he was sitting in the car glaring back at them, and shaking his fist.

"That is the very last time you will have to lay eyes on that creep, Shirley."

Will was aware that Shirley had been badly shaken by what had just happened.

Chapter Twenty Seven

"It's time to stop looking in the rear view mirror and start focusing on the road ahead." Unknown

"How many more spuds are left? I'm freezing out here."

Little Josie was eight years old and had peeled a stack of potatoes for lunch. It was her turn to be on vegetable peeling out in the lean-to. Everyone hated vegetable duty, but they all had to take their turn. Only the very little ones were excused.

"Still loads more. Sister said that we better hurry along or they won't get cooked in time."

Tom was trying to keep everyone in a positive frame of mind. He had learned a lot about morale in his nine years. His parents, had they lived, would have been very proud of him.

"I hate it in this shed. It's draughty and wet too, when the wind blows the rain in through the gaps. Why can't we peel the vegies in the kitchen? Sister keeps herself nice and warm in there with the stoves going."

Ella could always be relied on to speak her mind - as long as it was safe to do so.

"Sshhh. One of them may sneak up and hear you. Then we'll all cop it. Just shut up and get it done."

Johnnie was in charge of their little kitchen lackey team. He was eleven years old and he had been in St. Joseph's for five years, so he knew how to survive.

"Did you hear about Maxine and Theresa? Lucky things. They got the diphtheria and went to Northfield Hospital."

"Infectious Diseases Hospital. Get it right won't you."

Ruby was always particular about details. Little Josie (as she was always referred to, there being an older Josie) continued her story.

"Mary and Eric tried to catch it."

"How?" asked Muriel.

"Sister said that they should be very careful scrubbing out the milk churns, to get rid of the bacteria. She said that if they didn't take care, other children could catch diphtheria. So they licked the neck of the milk churns, hoping to catch that nasty disease. Then they would be able to go to the hospital."

All of the children listened and understood. They would give anything to escape St. Jo's for a time, even if it meant getting sick and going to hospital. Each day meant drudgery, deprivation, hunger, unkindness, punishment, threat, neglect and cruelty. Anything would be better than that.

"Is anyone else sick yet?"

Muriel was curious to hear. She pulled up the neck of her jumper, which was far too big for her, trying to keep out the cold. Her hands were wet and cold from peeling the spuds which were kept in a large tub of water.

"Wish they'd let us go back inside for a jacket. I didn't think it would be so cold today."

Muriel was shivering now.

"Hope I catch it. I'd love to have to stay indoors for awhile."

Johnnie nodded in agreement.

"Crabby black bats. I heard Shirley saying that her throat was very sore after breakfast. She looked very hot too. She'll be next. Lucky thing! It might cheer her up a bit. They say her stuttering started after they put her in prison here."

"Yeah. And it's been worse since she came back from that farm."

Ella looked down at her hands and sighed.

Someone to Watch Over Me

The children nodded in agreement and went on peeling potatoes with their knives, picking them up from the tubs of water and dropping them into stew pans when they were finished. The potatoes were unwashed and the children had to brush off the dirt before peeling them. The dirt got under their fingernails and everywhere it wanted to settle. They all knew that Sister Beatrice (the nun in charge of the kitchen) would pounce at any time, like the cat on the poor mouse. Talking was not allowed in "The Shed." It was seen as a distraction from the work that the children had to get done.

However, they kept up their spirits by defying some of the unrealistic demands, and when they were at work in "the Shed" they took turns in being the sentry, watching out for horrid Sister Beatrice. Much gossip was shared this way, and the distraction actually helped them to get the work done more swiftly.

"Poor Shirley said she's scared of eating in the dining room now. She said there are heaps more rats that come out from the skirting boards and eat the scraps off the floor than were there before. She is very scared of the rats."

Ella hated them too and was very nervous that they would come out of their hiding places before she had finished her meal and left the table.

"I'm not scared of any silly rats. If they come near me I'll kick them with my shoe."

Johnnie's bravado was not challenged as the girl's liked to have someone in their group who might protect them even if it was out of his need to be seen as strong and courageous.

Chapter Twenty Eight

"The greater part of our happiness or misery depends on our dispositions and not on our circumstances." Martha Washington

Shirley Gilfillan was ecstatic! She had just seen the doctor, and he had looked at her throat and felt her glands in her neck. She held her breath as she waited for his verdict. It seemed as if he would never speak.

"I'm sorry to say that this little one has diphtheria too, and must go immediately to hospital. It is a very contagious disease, so we must move her urgently, before anyone else has a chance to catch it. It seems to be going through your home like a packet of Epsom Salts. You need to look at your hygiene and make some drastic changes."

His concerns about the children caused him to find courage and his words were a slap in the face to Sister Gertrude. The prickly nun raised herself in her chair, squaring her shoulders and looking as superior as she could, she growled at the "audacious" doctor.

"There is nothing at all wrong with our hygiene, Doctor" she sniffed.

Shirley almost giggled at the exchange. Nothing would spoil her excitement at this news. Escape at last. This was a chance to get out of this horrible place for a time at least. Maybe weeks, if she was lucky. Forgetting the doctor's instructions, she ran from the sick room to find her friends. He darted out of the door after her, but he was not fast enough. Standing outside the door waiting to hear her best friend's news was Rita.

"R-r-rita. I've g-g-got it. H-h-here, let me b-b-breathe on you and y-you might be l-lucky too."

Shirley's joy was evident and her intention obvious as she put her face right in front of Rita's and breathed out as hard as she could.

Before Rita could say a word, the doctor grabbed Shirley, chastising her as he made her return to the sick room off the dormitory. The priest was called and he quickly marched her to his car and then transported her to the Northfield Infectious Diseases Hospital, situated on Hampstead Road and just over six miles from the Royal Adelaide Hospital in the city of Adelaide.

The Northfield Hospital had been opened in 1932 to provide care for people with such diseases as poliomyelitis, scarlet fever, measles and diphtheria. Dr. McIntosh knew that in 1934, ten of the patients who were admitted with diphtheria had died. It was now 1937 and they were in the middle of a diphtheria epidemic. It was most common where people lived in crowded situations, so he was not surprised that it had broken out in St. Joseph's Orphanage.

Dr. McIntosh also knew that the disease was passed on through close contact and he was aware that the hygiene in the orphanage was not always as he would like. He was very worried about a dangerous outbreak with some of the children dying from the disease.

He frowned as he counted the growing number of infected children who had been transported to the Northfield Hospital, from St. Joseph's Orphanage.

Shirley loved the ride to the hospital, and relished the country scenery that the hospital nestled in. There were paddocks around it and the sky was a pretty blue with the clouds making a fluffy white contrast and looking like bunny tails. Her heart skipped as she gazed at the colours of freedom.

Someone to Watch Over Me

The "House of Horrors" was behind her, and her life was about to change. She had heard from the other children who had come here that it was a good place. If she was lucky, she would take weeks to get well.

Please Lord Jesus, please don't let me get well for a very long time, she thought.

The dormitory only held a few beds, not like the orphanage dormitory which held twenty five or more. To her amazement, there was a radio on a shelf. She clapped her hands and jumped up and down on the spot. Music. How wonderful. The sheets were white and crisp and the pillows plump and soft. She had a little cupboard alongside her bed. She knew it was probably empty because she had nothing to bring and they had left in a hurry. It was hers anyway, and that felt good. Something that she could call her own.

The warm and sunny nurse floated into the room like she had butterfly wings. She wore a white uniform with a scarf thing on her hair. Shirley could see her blond curls struggling to get away from their containment. She also noticed the twinkle in the kindly blue eyes.

What a beautiful place, thought the eleven year old. She smiled sweetly at the nurse and stood very still until she was told to move. Just like in "the home."

"Well, what a cute one you are Shirley. And how polite. We'll have to keep those boys locked in their room down the corridor. They'll all want to come check out the new girl. And what pretty manners. Come along now and we'll get you into a gown and into bed. Do you know any of these girls in your room? I think most of them are from St. Joseph's aren't they? Yes, that's right. You are all part of the big family there so you are going to get along really well."

The chatty nurse was working while she was speaking, going from bed to bed and checking each child in her travels, having

Someone to Watch Over Me

drawn a curtain around Shirley's bed after she placed a gown on top of her candlewick bedspread.

Very quickly Shirley was standing alongside her bed, in her white hospital gown and looking like a little angel, complete with cheeks blushing a rosy pink. (Even if the colour was from her high temperature). Nurse swished back the curtain, and the new patient decided that she loved the sound.

"Don't worry about nurse, Shirley. She says that to all the new girls. You are going to love it here. The nurses are so kind and the food is nothing like the pig slops at St. Jo's. And we don't have to "earn our keep." They have people who get paid to do all the hard work. We are having a holiday and don't ever want to get well. We get to choose our programmes on the radio too. And we get to go outside to play in the paddocks, when we feel a bit better."

Shirley stared at Hannah. She recognised her as one of the older girls who hardly ever spoke at the orphanage. Here she was, talking away like a real chatterbox.

"Yesterday some of us went outside to play and I made daisy chains from the dandelions. Mine was the longest. Nurse told me I'm very good with my hands. She is going to get someone to show me how to embroider. She thinks I would be very good at it."

Shirley recognised Hilda and smiled to see how chirpy she had become. She was such a sad little tyke where they all came from, but now her spirit was alive and cheerful. Her enthusiasm gave Shirley hope for good times ahead. She lay on her bed and quickly nodded off into a much needed sleep.

She was mortified. There was blood on her sheet. It was on the back of her gown and her legs felt sticky. She must be very sick. The diphtheria must be spreading throughout her body. She was going to die. Shirley started to cry, bursting into tears with her face in her hands.

"Whatever is the matter, Shirley Whirley?"

Someone to Watch Over Me

Hannah was the first to jump out of her bed and race to her. Before long she had several girls standing around her and looking at her bed and her gown. Looks passed from girl to girl and then a couple of them started to laugh. Soon there was a chorus of tinkling laughter, and Shirley stopped crying, curious as to why her friends would think it so funny that she was going to die.

"That's just your "girlfriend," said Bernadette.

"You are not dying" said Hilda. "You're growing up. Nurse told me all about it when it happened to Meg. She was upset too, and nurse fixed her up in no time."

Shirley slowly caught on and stopped crying. She had heard about this but didn't think it would happen to her for years. She was only eleven for goodness sake. She thought it was something to do with having babies and she sure didn't want one of those until she was really old, like twenty one, and married. She suddenly thought of Carrieton and tried to make herself forget, thanking Jesus and crossing herself as she did that she didn't have her "girlfriend" back then. She shuddered when she realised how lucky she was that she didn't get a baby from that horrible old man. Tears filled her eyes and she wrapped her arms around herself, trying to bring comfort as the ugly memories terrorised her.

Hannah gave her a quick hug and then rang the little bell that sat on her cupboard.

"Don't move Shirley. Nurse will clean you up and give you something to put on and then she'll fix your bed. You don't have to do anything. Nurse will do it for you. Isn't it wonderful how they treat us here? Don't be upset sweetie. Everything will be taken care of and you won't get told off or punished (or pinched) either."

Shirley had told no-one of her experiences at Carrieton. When she arrived back at St. Joseph's with the social worker, the nuns said nothing to her of her ordeal. No questions were asked. No comfort was given. Everything went on just as before. The religious women, who called themselves "the brides of Christ," seemed blind to her broken spirit and showed no compassion for her deep heartache. Nevertheless there was an upside as their neglect enabled her to try to put the whole experience behind her and to throw herself into the events of each day.

But deep down in the dungeon of her soul, dark shadows lurked behind a heavy padlocked door.

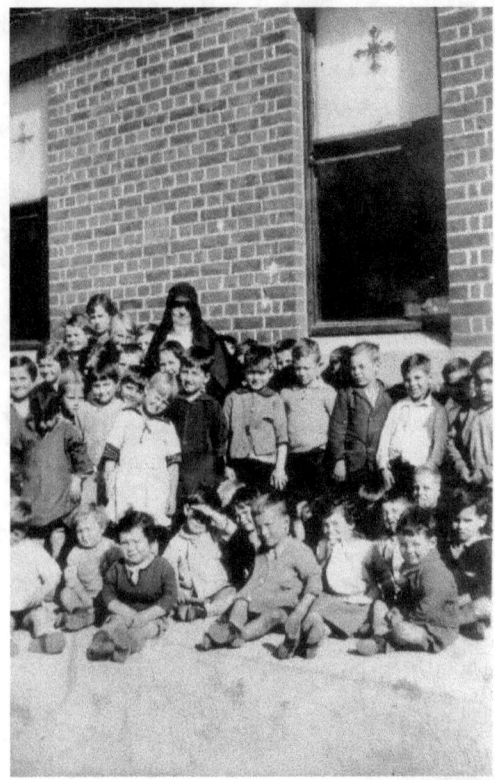

Only childhood photo of Shirley. Taken at St. Joseph's Catholic Orphanage. Shirley is on the left in second row from top.

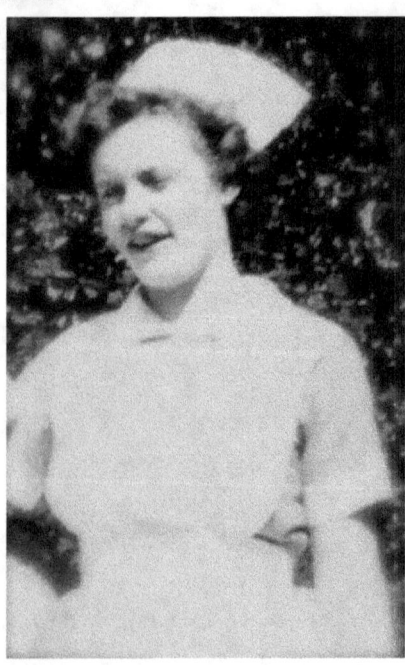

Shirley at Ru Rua Hospital in her nurse's aid uniform at 15 years

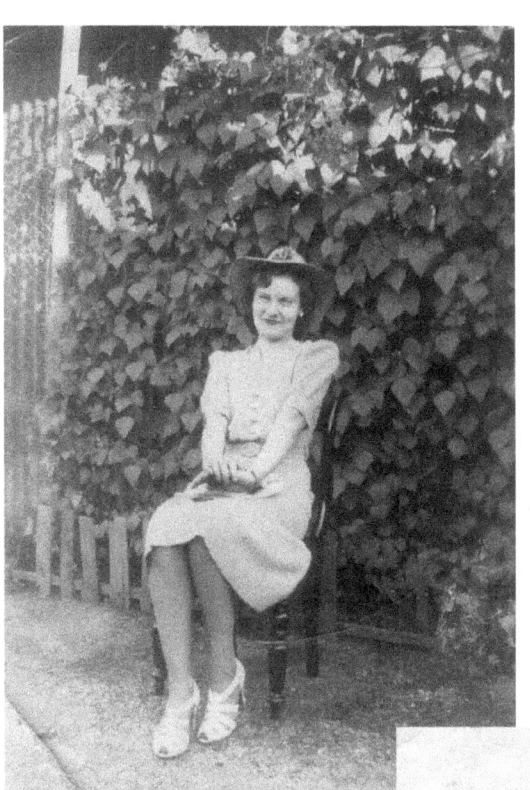

Sweet sixteen

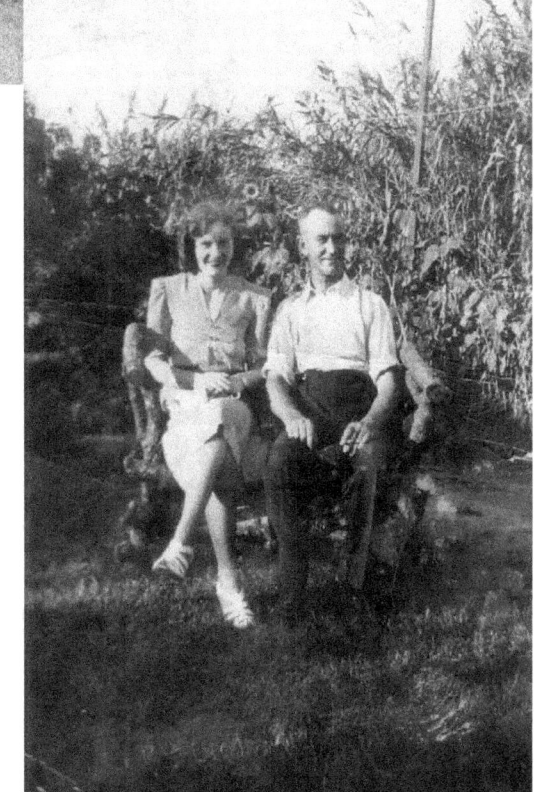

Shortly after Shirley was reunited with her father, Percy Gilfillan

Recapturing a missed childhood

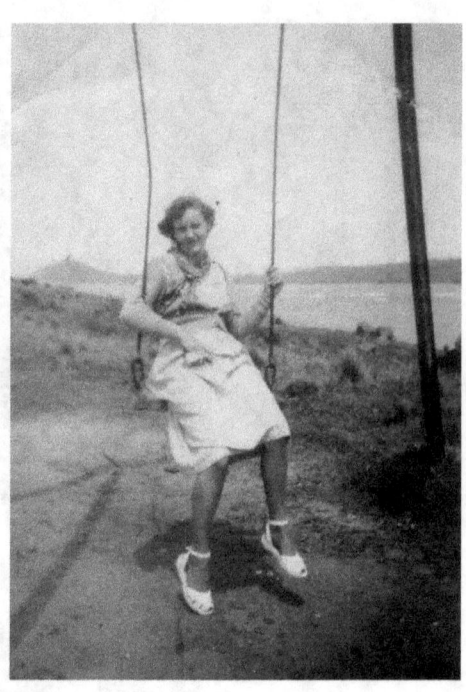

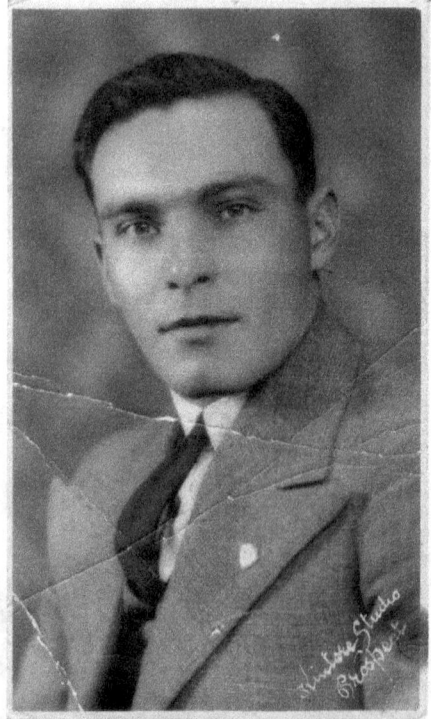

Burton James Clough about the time he met Shirley

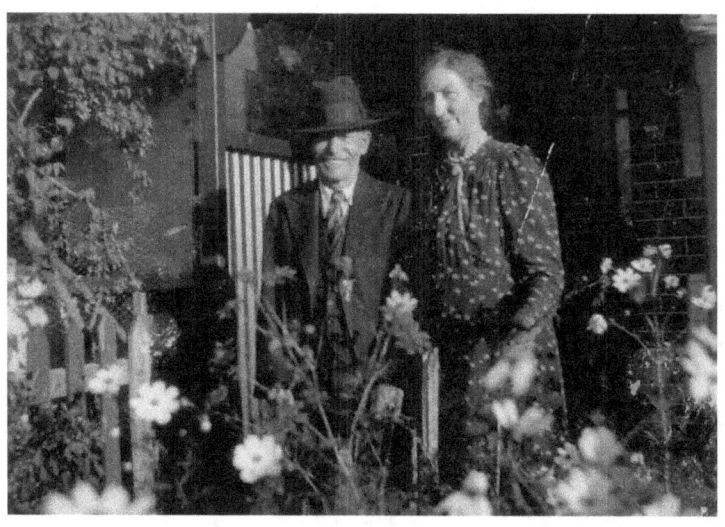

Burt's parents, Walter and Margaret Clough

Engaged

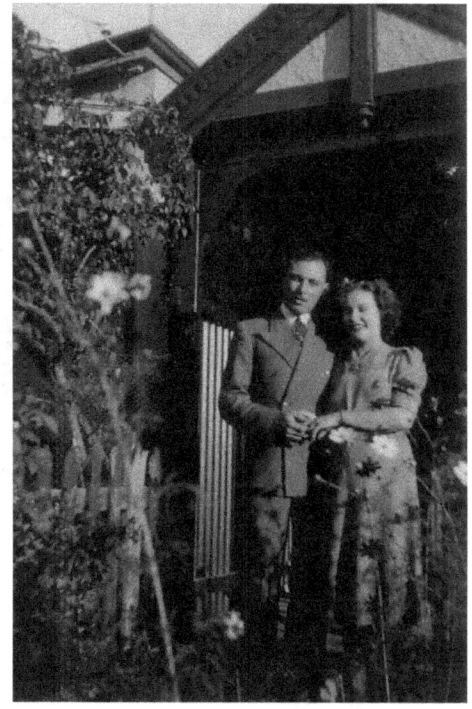

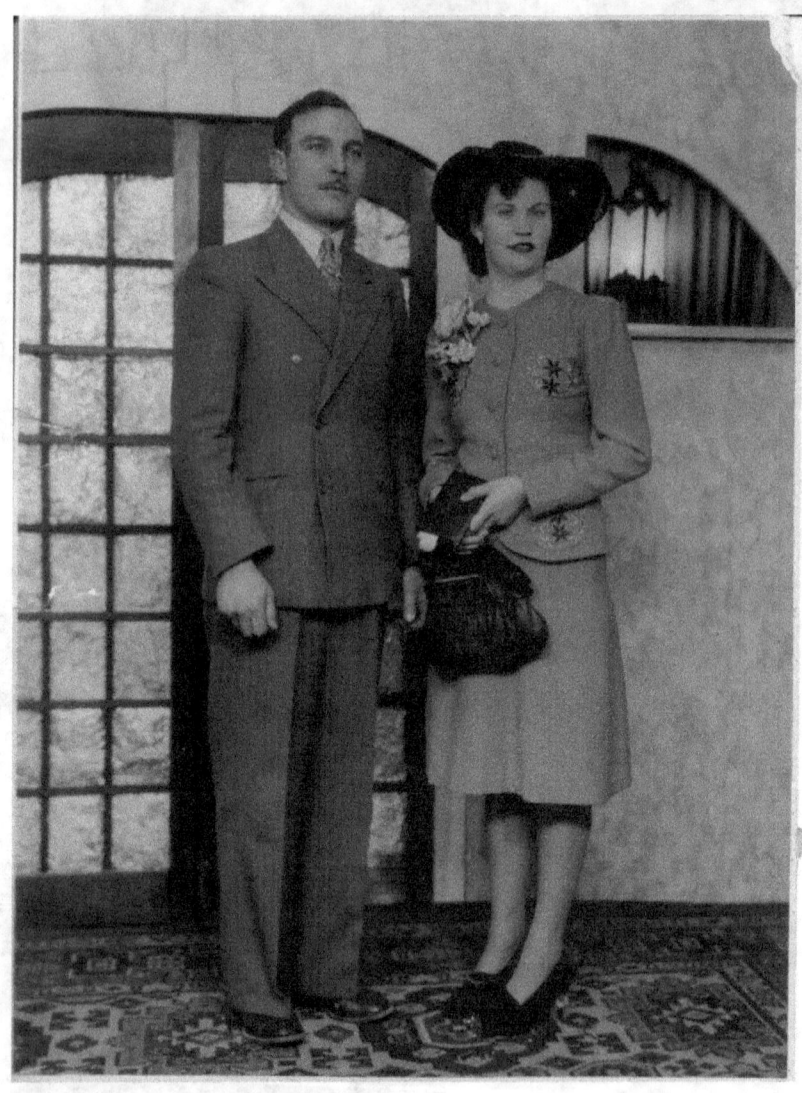

Shirley and Burt's Wedding Day

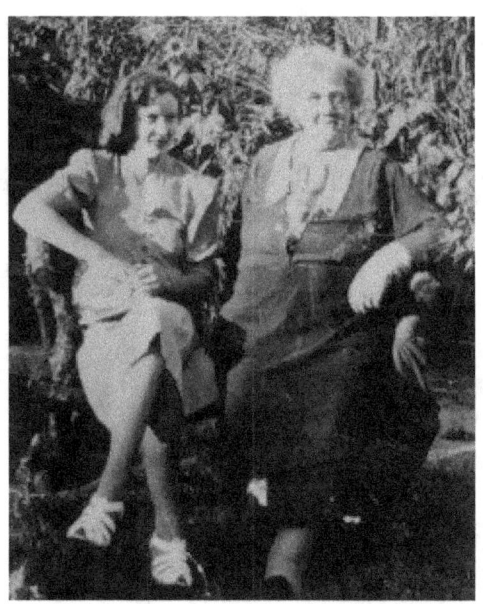

Shirley with her beloved Mrs Nora M. Noonan – a mother and a grandmother in the same package

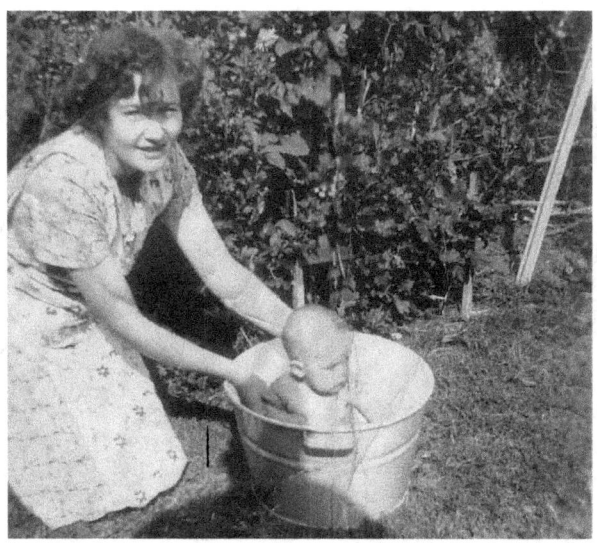

Shirley with baby Patricia

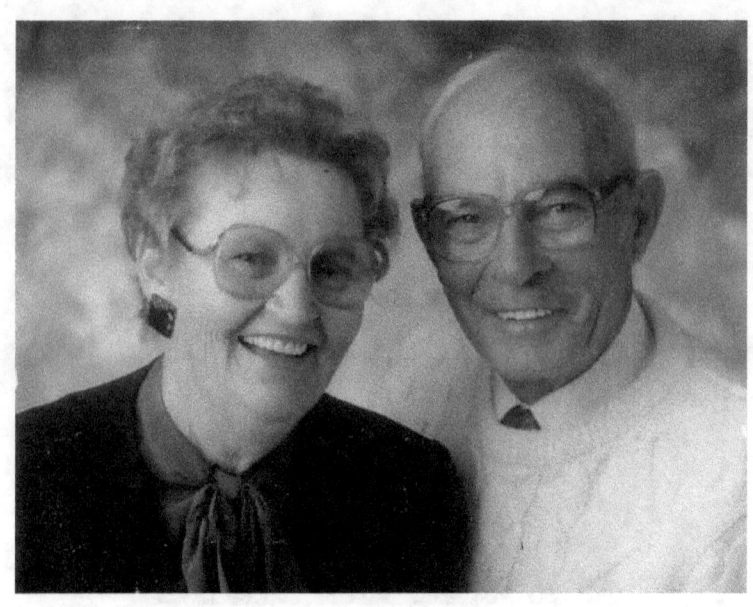

Above and below: Celebrating fifty years of marriage

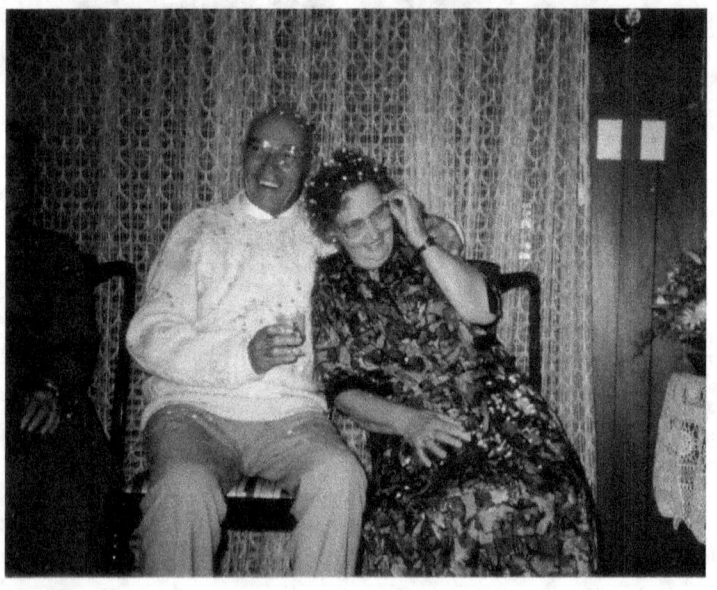

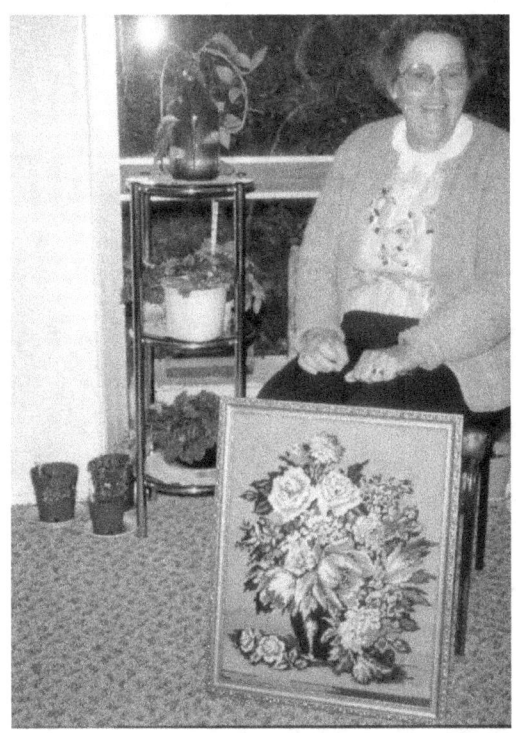

One of her many tapestries – a challenge with only one eye

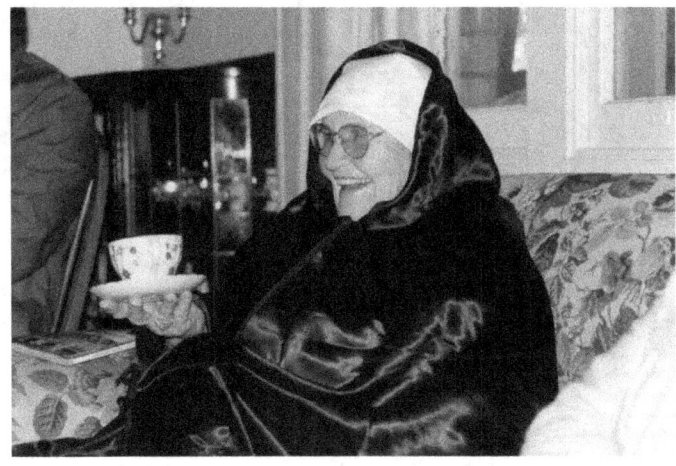

Making peace with the past in fancy dress

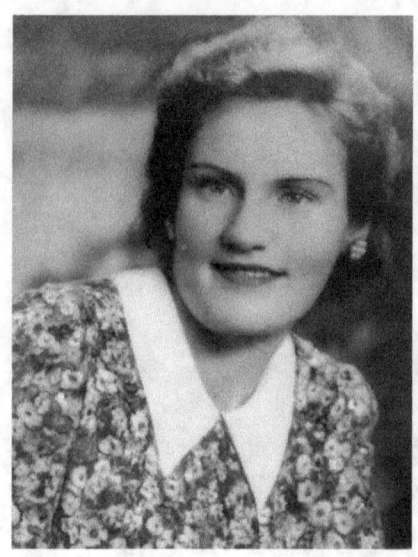

Shirley in her favourite dress – her maternity dress for six babies

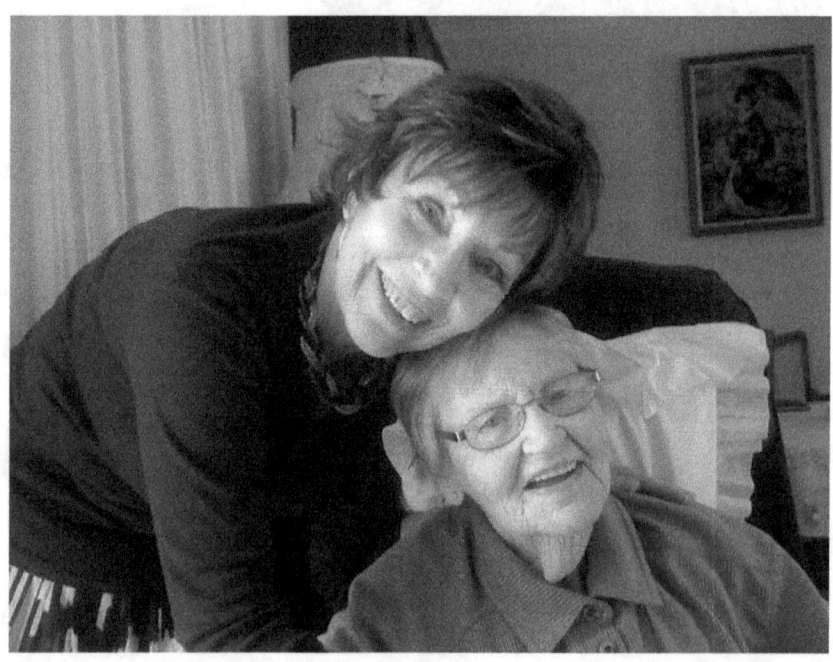

The author with her mother

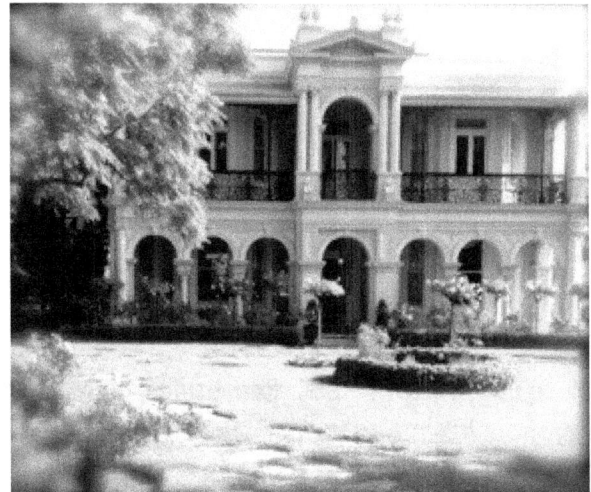

Audley House on Prospect Road, where Shirley worked as a fifteen year old live-in maid for the Lawrences

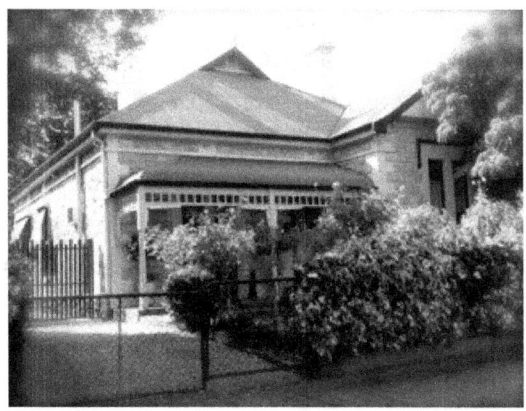

The Noonan's house in Prospect where Shirley went into service at eleven years of age

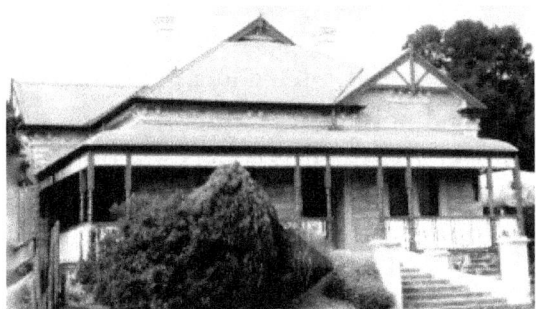

The Brogan's house where Shirley was a live-in maid and met Burt Clough

Chapter Twenty Nine

"Never be afraid to try something new. Remember, amateurs built the Ark, professionals built the Titanic." Author Unknown

Three blissful months had passed at "the hospital" and Shirley had become accustomed to "Heaven" as the children had nick-named their oasis. Most of the nurses were angels and there was white everywhere. The doctors were kind and the cooks loved to have a good laugh.

She had been there for a lot longer than usual because the doctor could not get a "clear swab" of her throat. Shirley knew in her heart that her prayers to Jesus had worked. She did not tell anyone though because she had told one of the girls once and she had screwed up her nose in derision. This was Shirley's secret and she would keep praying and see if she could stay for another three months.

Sometimes she felt like being a little girl and day-dreaming and so she did. Other times she would remember some of the awful things from her past and get upset and angry. She would sit and brood and the black feeling would settle like a heavy cape around her head and shoulders. Sometimes she would decide to be happy and shrug off the memories, pretending to be someone else. Some young girl who had nothing at all that was dark and menacing in her past. When she thought of Charlie and how badly she missed him, Shirley quickly dismissed the thought, pretending that she had never known someone by that name. Some of the children had visitors and received letters or cards.

Someone to Watch Over Me

Shirley was jealous. No-one remembered her or made any contact with her. Three whole months in hospital and she had heard from no-one. What had happened to her father? Where was her grandmother? Why did her mother not even send a note or a card? Where had Charlie gone?

The thoughts flittered back into her mind like butterflies on gossamer wings. No! They were more like ugly black bats sweeping into a dark cave and screeching for attention. Shirley's mind was all over the place, keeping pace with her jumbled emotions. She tried to forget. She screwed up her face, trying to remember what her mother looked like. Her mother, who was in a hospital too. Not a nice mother. Shirley quickly pretended that she was not her real mother. She was just a crazy woman that her own mother knew. Her own mother would be kind and sweet and bring flowers and lollies and she would sit on her bed and read her stories, and stroke her hair and call her "sweetie" and darling." Her real mother would never make her eye blind and hit her and hurt her and say cruel words to her. She would think of a nice mother that she wished she had. She must not think of how cruel her own mother had been. She would think of someone who would be a lovely mother to wish for. Like Mrs. Bennett. Dear, kind, Mrs. Bennett who brought her a salty rag for her sore face when she was all alone on her bed, sick with mumps. Mrs. Bennett, who bathed her forehead and patted her hand when she cried for Charlie. Charlie who? She didn't know a Charlie. Don't think about him. He doesn't care. Think about Mrs. Bennett, yes, she was kind. *She loved me* thought the lonely child, lonely and pining to be cared about and remembered and loved.

She broke down, sobbing into her pillow. Nurse Miriam came and sat on her bed and stroked her hair.

"What is it Shirley. What has upset you?"

Shirley blurted out the thoughts that had been tormenting her and the kindly nurse listened intently. When she had finished, the nurse jumped up from the bed and disappeared for a moment or two, arriving back with some note paper, a pencil and an envelope.

"Here, Shirley Whirley. You write a nice letter to that kind neighbour of yours who looked after you with your mumps. I will post it and before you know it, I bet she comes to see you, or sends you a letter back."

Nancy, in the bed alongside Shirley's bed noticed with surprise, that nurse had one hand behind her back, with her fingers crossed.

The address was unknown to the girl so nurse suggested that she address it to Mrs. Bennett of Cowandilla and someone might know her and make sure that she received it. Nurse Miriam's confidence fired up Shirley. She spent a long time over her letter, painstakingly spelling out each word with the girls in the neighbouring beds. She knew that she was not good at writing or spelling but she tried anyway. It was a heartfelt attempt to manage at least one visit from anyone while she was in hospital.

"Dear Mrs. Bennett,

I am your little neighbour Shirley. I am 11 now. I am in hospital and I hope I can stay here for a very long time. It is nice here. The only thing wrong is that no-one ever comes to see me. It is alright though because the nurses are my friends. The girls here are my friends too. I get sad when they have to go back to St. Joseph's Orphanage though. It is not good there. I wish I never had to go back there.

I should be grateful. At least they took us in, when no-one else wanted us. I wonder where Charlie is and why he doesn't come to see me. I don't know where my Daddy is. My granny hasn't been to see me either. They must all be very busy. It is a long way out here, nurse says.

Someone to Watch Over Me

My "swabs" are never clear so I just keep staying here. My prayers are answered. I am also praying for a visitor. Do you think God is interested in my prayers? I do, because my swabs are never clear.

I remember often how kind you were to me when I was so scared and sad on my own, with the mumps. Thank you for bringing the salty rag. I hope you and your family are happy. It must be lovely to have a family.

I hope I get to see you again one day.
Love
Shirley"

Shirley sat on her bed, wishing she had her photo of Jesus to pray to.

Please Lord Jesus. Let Mrs. Bennett come to see me.

The sunny nurse collected her letter, folding it and placing it in the envelope.

"Miracles happen, Shirley. Never ever give up."

Chapter Thirty

"Wherever I go today help me leave heartprints!
Heartprints of compassion, of understanding and love."
Unknown

It was raining outside and a cold front had pushed its way in. Everyone had been rugged up inside for a couple of days and Shirley and her friends were lying on their beds talking amongst themselves. Her other friends had all dribbled back to St. Josephs one after the other, but new girls kept coming and replacing them.

Someone was standing in the doorway. A woman. A stranger. The girls all looked at each other with a silent question. Shoulders shrugged and eyebrows raised. Each girl wanted the stranger to be their very own visitor. Someone to make them feel important and remembered. Presents were not even thought about. Just someone who liked them enough to come.

Silence hung in the ward. Everyone waited for the stranger to speak and reveal her identity. She was a nice looking woman. She had on a grey suit and a perky dark pink hat. On her hands she wore black leather gloves and in them she carried a black "clutch" bag. Her feet looked pretty in black high heeled shoes. Finally the silence was broken.

"Who is Shirley?"

Everything seemed to go into slow motion for the girl whose name had just been mentioned. Everyone was looking at her. Envy on their faces.

"I-I am," said Shirley, from her bed. She was too afraid to move and break the spell. Was this a dream? Had someone really come to visit her? Her? Shirley Gilfillan? The forgotten. The unwanted.

"My name is Mrs. Bennett," said the stranger. She opened her clutch bag and took out a letter. The lovely lady walked graciously over to the bed of the child who had just spoken and asked if she had sent the letter.

"Y-y-yes Mrs. B-Bennett," said Shirley, as if she had done something wrong. She hung her head, afraid the lady would realise that she did not recognise the child and disappear.

"You touched my heart, Shirley. I could tell that you were a lovely girl, and I badly wanted to come and meet you. It was a beautiful letter. I have read it many times and want to congratulate you on being such a clever girl to think of sending it and getting me to visit."

She stopped speaking for a moment as she saw the tears rolling down the face of the lonely child.

"I think you must have meant another Mrs. Bennett, but I was the lucky Mrs. Bennett who received your letter. I hope you are not too disappointed and that I will do."

All of the girls were staring. Hardly breathing. Mouths open wide and silent. Shirley's pretty face was aglow. Her eyes blue and shiny with tears.

"Y-yes. You will do....I-I mean....I d-don't mean it like that....you w-will MORE than do...thank you....thank y-you."

She was crying now with joy, and words were choking in her throat.

"Here Shirley. I have this pretty hanky that I brought just for you. It looks like you need it right now. Also, I have a book that you might like to read. Here it is...."

Shirley's new friend took it carefully out of her bag and handed it to the weeping girl.

"It looks lovely.......a-a-and the p-print is j-just the right size. I have a bit of trouble reading. E-especially if the p-print is small and there is l-lots of it," said the child with shame.

"It is a story of a brave young girl who has some hard things in her life. She rises above her troubles and becomes a brilliant and famous singer. She reminds me of how brave you are."

"Shirley's a great singer," said Therese. "She sings to us all sometimes and she has a lovely voice. Her grandmother sang on the stage. She takes after her, nurse says."

Mrs. Bennett turned back to Shirley with admiration on her face.

"It seems I bought just the right book, dear, without knowing about your lovely voice. Do you think you would sing for me one day? I would love to hear you."

The happy girl nodded her head slowly and deliberately. Her face beamed with the promise of a new friendship and more visits to come.

Someone to Watch Over Me

Chapter Thirty One

"Where is the good in goodbye"

Meredith Wilson. The Music Man

Eventually the inevitable day came and Shirley's swab was clear. She had to return to St. Jo's. When she received the news, the young girl broke down with disappointment. It was as if the lights had gone out for her. She begged and pleaded, promised and prayed. She sobbed and sulked. It was hopeless. She had to go back.

Northfield Infectious Diseases Hospital had been a place of sunshine and music. Her Mrs. Bennet (the new Mrs. Bennet) had been to visit her several times. They had become great friends. Shirley had been very game one day and bravely asked if Mrs. Bennet could adopt her. There had been no shock or negative reaction on the lady's face, only sadness as she said how much she would love to do this, but it would not be allowed as she was Protestant and not Catholic. This had to do for the child. To know that Mrs. Bennet would have loved to if she could have.

Her visitor brought her little gifts and also something for the other girls in the ward to share. She was the best visitor any little girl in hospital could ever wish for. Jesus had heard her prayers and had answered her so wonderfully. He was real and He cared. He would help her to cope at St. Josephs. She would pray and He would give her the strength to endure.

Her goodbyes to her friends at the hospital were almost too much for her to bear. Even her doctor came out to the priest's car to see her off. The nurses hugged her and wished her well. So did the girls from her ward who were crying as they said goodbye. Someone gave her a tiny bunch of violets from the garden and another gave her a pencil and a notebook to write in.

"Keep up that practice with your writing, Shirl. You have improved a great deal. All you need is practice. That is all. You are a bright young lady," said her favourite nurse. The tears flowed for the grateful girl.

Shirley hid the violets under her jacket and the pencil in her pocket. Her notebook went up under her dress and into the top of her panties, at the back. She had learned the hard way to hide anything that was given to her, away from the sight and clutches of the nasty women in black.

Someone to Watch Over Me

Chapter Thirty Two

"Only in the agony of parting do we look into the depths of love." George Eliot

The girls giggled as they told their stories to each other. They were in the bathroom and it was Friday night (confession night). They all had to go into the confession box, one by one and tell the priest their sins, and receive absolution. It became a game to see who could make up the best story. Their greatest "sin" was lying to the priest as they were expected to "confess" something and he wouldn't let them go until they had.

"I told him that I took two lollies instead of our one a year that Mrs. O'Grady always gets for us on St. Patrick's Day," piped up the strong and defiant Jacinta.

"I told him that I wouldn't hold hands when we walked in pairs to the Semaphore pictures," said her competitive sister Muriel.

Not to be outdone, Shirley chirped,

"I told him that I lied when I said that I liked "Alexander's Ragtime Band." I didn't lie really. I loved the picture. The music was wonderful. It was good tricking him though. I don't like him. He's mean."

All the children loved their occasional walks to the picture theatre. It was a huge highlight for all of them in their deprivation.

"At least they get the old projector out of the cupboard now and again and show us a movie. The stupid priest still can't work it properly and the movie keeps jumping and stopping. He's better than hopeless sister Francesca, though. She can never work out which is the turn on switch."

Jacinta was getting very game in their secluded moment of sharing and giggling.

"Well, I was the best of all," said Betty. "I told him that I sneaked a look at the boys at the beach when we went the other day. I wonder if he even knows that they have to go so far down the beach from us that I would need binoculars to see the boys!"

They fell all over each other, laughing and escaping the tension for awhile.

It was time once again for farewell. Shirley's friends gathered again in the quadrangle. Goodbyes were unbearable and all too frequent in her young life. This was one thing that did not get better with experience.

Her gang of girls had welcomed her back with enthusiasm when she had finally returned from the Northfield Infectious Diseases Hospital. Upon her return, she had been summoned to sister's office. Sister Gertrude asked her if she was well enough to go as live-in help to an old couple in Prospect. Shirley felt a shock wave go through her tiny body. It was as if a team of draught horses were dragging her off in different directions. She was afraid, she was sad about leaving her friends and the familiar, she was nervous about whether the couple would like her and if she could measure up to their expectations, she wondered if she would find young friends in Prospect and she felt a flicker of excitement in her chest.

"Yes," she was well enough.

Was that the only criteria? Was it safe for an eleven year old girl? Was the work too heavy for a child? Were the people kind? Would she be looked after? Would she have any free time? Would there ever be opportunity for fun? How would she get to meet other young ones her own age? So many questions she wanted to ask, but experience had taught her that it was best to keep silent.

"Good then. You will have a day or two while they get ready for you. Start getting your things together. Select a couple of things from the clean laundry basket. You may like to take a coat as the weather is getting cold. Off you go then. I think cook is expecting you in the kitchen to assist her. There are some extra guests for lunch and she needs your help."

It was time. The priest had his car ready and the moment of departure had come. Shirley hugged and kissed her friends goodbye once more. Little Bobby came running up and nearly bowled her over with a very enthusiastic hug. A tear somehow escaped and cascaded down her cheek.

"Look after yourself Bobby. You are such a good boy and your life will turn around. Don't give up hope. Remember to say your prayers. And don't suck those middle fingers. That way the sisters won't have anything to pick on you about."

She was crying openly now. The emotions tumbled over her and her throat ached as she fought back the tears. Slowly looking into each face that belonged to her adopted family, memories washed over her. She wondered if this was the last time she would ever be at St. Jo's and if she would ever see her dear friends again.

Her best friend Rita was crying also. Struggling with her own sadness, Shirley tried to think of something comforting to say to the girl who had been the sister that she never had.

"Look after Bobby for me Rita. You are the only one that I would trust him to."

Rita nodded her head, unable to speak.

The insensitive priest hurried her along and she climbed into his old jalopy, which was bound for a place she had never been before, Prospect, and an unknown future.

Someone to Watch Over Me

As the car bounced through the gateway, she looked at the small gathering of friends who sadly waved her goodbye and good luck.

These are my family, she thought to herself. *These are the ones who have suffered with me and who truly love me. I love them too and will miss them more than anything.*

Chapter Thirty Three

"Life is ten percent what happens to us and ninety percent how we respond to it." Albert M. Wells Jr.

The adolescent sat silently in the back seat. The scenery hurried past as she watched out of the window with eyes that did not see. Tears welled and blurred the view. Feelings overwhelmed her and her face was awash as scalding tears hurried down her cheeks, pooling on her chin.

Why am I crying? she asked herself, brushing angrily at the offensive show of emotion. *Nothing bad has happened today to make me cry. What a sook I am. I should be thankful that someone is willing to take me in and give me a chance.*

She wiped her face with her sleeve and wiped her leaky nose with the back of her hand. Reaching down she grabbed the tired and badly creased grey skirt, lifting it towards her face, to mop up the remaining dampness. She struggled to hold in the sobs that kept trying to escape, saying to herself over and over again, *Stop it. Stop it. Stop it.*

As she watched through the window, the passing housing styles and gardens looked more and more attractive. She noticed the tree-lined streets and the care that was taken in the yards.

Hope rose on wings in her chest. Before long they reached their destination in Prospect. The priest found the house without too much trouble, and pulled up in front of a rather grand looking home. The garden was full of splashes of colour from rose and lavender bushes that had a mind of their own and pretty daisies of white and pink, with a large bird of paradise plant that looked magnificent, as it pretended to be a green and leafy plant with a display of colourful birds sitting on its leaves. Shady trees and leafy shrubs of various colours of green scattered across the front garden. The house was a stylish Villa with a bull nose veranda, showing off an attractive timber decorative trim, and tall chimneys with a promise of warmth in winter. There were statues and a bird bath to decorate and charm. The garden sang a friendly welcome as Shirley drank in the colour and beauty.

Then she noticed the three wheeler bike on the front veranda. Sister Cecilia had told her that Mrs. Nora Noonan had something wrong with her legs and that she rode her bike when she went to the shops, rather than walk. Kindly Cecilia had encouraged her anxious heart, explaining that Mrs. Noonan was a very nice lady and would be kind to the young girl, and that Mr. Thomas Noonan was a good man who was honourable and kind.

Nicer than the unfriendly priest who had just driven her for many miles with hardly a word spoken. Not a word of encouragement or comfort to the young girl. Not even a joke to laugh about.

"We're here. Out you get."

Why do these people who have no idea of how to treat children get to be in charge of us? Shirley was growing up and questioning the injustices of her environment.

A huge lady with a round face, a long string of pearls, a flowery dress, and with small glasses perched on the end of her nose, appeared in the doorway, a welcoming smile on her friendly face.

"Well, here you are at last. You must be Shirley."

Her large frame matched her very big voice. Sister Cecilia had told her that Mr. and Mrs. Noonan had been farmers at one time and that Mrs. Noonan had also worked as a high school teacher. At one stage the teacher had opened the school at Booborowie and taught there for eight years.

She took a keen interest in young people, encouraging numbers of them in their careers. When the Noonans retired, they moved from the Gulnare district to Adelaide, where Mrs. Noonan was well known for her hospitality and charity work.

"H-h-hello Mrs. Noonan," said Shirley, curtseying and keeping her eyes down, as if she was meeting royalty.

"Oh my goodness. No need for any of that sort of thing around here child. If we end up liking each other, you will be one of the family." The kindly woman knew how to educate any newcomer very quickly, to the lay of the land.

"Hello Father. I hope you didn't find the trip too arduous and that my instructions were precise. Being country folk originally, Mr. Noonan and I are better at mud maps than following directories."

She smiled at the priest as she spoke.

"Thank you Mrs. Noonan, your instructions were very clear indeed. We came straight here with no mishaps or wrong turns whatsoever."

Father O'Rourke was anxious to keep his orphanage supporter happy. He knew that the Noonans were reasonably well-off and that they had been generous to St. Josephs in the past.

"Come along inside and let me find something for you to eat and drink. The kettle is on and I am sure that you would both enjoy a nice cup of tea."

The accommodating hostess ushered the priest and young girl in through her front door and invited them to take a seat in her tastefully furnished sitting room.

Shirley felt most uncomfortable as she was feeling that she should be waiting on everyone else and not being treated like a special visitor. She sat on the edge of her seat on the settee, as if she was expecting to jump up at any moment.

"Just sit back and relax child. There will be plenty for you to do when the time comes. The 'help' whose name is Mrs. Dorsey is in the kitchen and she will bring in tea for us in just a moment."

Mrs. Noonan picked up a small china bell from her sideboard and shook it gently. It tinkled like a fairy bell and "the help" appeared immediately, wiping her hands on her apron and smiling a huge and warm welcome to Shirley, who could not believe her luck. For the first time in her life, she was eating delicious cake with a polished silver cake fork, and from a delicate bone china cake plate. The cake was a sponge that was as light as a feather and there was a vanilla custard filling with a homemade mock raspberry jam in the centre. It was crowned with a rich butter icing that had been coloured baby pink. She ate every crumb and her eyes kept straying back to the large cake plate with the pretty pink roses, which matched her own small plate. On it sat the remainder of the cake, inviting her to have another piece. She licked her lips, imagining the delicacy melting in her mouth.

"No use keeping a sponge as left-overs. I will be offended if you do not have another piece. I am well known in Prospect for my afternoon teas and I would be greatly disappointed if you did not tuck in and enjoy seconds."

Mrs. Noonan had noticed Shirley's eyes wandering back to the left-over cake and was determined that the skinny child would have her fill. She knew, intuitively, that this would not occur until others were served seconds first of all.

Very quickly, seconds were handed around, the priest leading with his extended plate, and the little group enjoying their delicious treat. Shirley had a look of absolute bliss as she savoured the cool, smooth, custard on her palate and allowed the tart taste of mock raspberry jam to tickle her unpracticed taste buds.

Glancing at his watch, Father O'Rourke excused himself and took his leave, somehow forgetting to say "goodbye" to the "package" he had delivered. The hostess saw him out of her front door, farewelled him and then turned to Shirley, winked and exclaimed, "At last. I thought he'd never go. Now I can show you your new home."

When shown to her own room, Shirley was speechless. She had never seen anything so exquisitely lovely before in her whole life. There were pretty lavender curtains at her window and her quilt on her white painted bed matched beautifully. On the quilt sat a celluloid baby doll, in a delicate hand knitted ice blue baby outfit. It was knitted in a fancy lacy pattern and the doll-deprived girl longed to pick it up and cuddle it. The room had little touches here and there that made it look like that of any ordinary and much loved young girl. Tears rushed to her eyes as she noticed the pretty mat on the polished wood floor, near her bed for comfort, and the books arranged on her dressing table. Mrs. Noonan had a new brush and some ribbons for her hair and also some talcum powder with a picture of roses on the front. Best of all, there was a gift there, all wrapped up in pretty paper and tied with a lavender ribbon.

Shirley was embarrassed and tried not to notice the gift. Her eyes kept going back to it until finally Mrs. Noonan spoke up.

"Well, aren't you going to see what it is?"

"W-would that be alright i-if I d-d-did?"

"Go on, I want to see if you like it, girl." Mrs. Noonan had been standing in the doorway watching the excited child, and was delighted to see her joy.

Shirley quickly and carefully unwrapped the gift, her hands shaking as she did so. There was a second layer of tissue paper which caused the gift to seem even more precious. Slowly she unwrapped the last layer. Her eyes were shiny with joy and she could not speak because her throat felt funny and no words would come. Inside the tissue sat a purple, velvet box and inside the box sat a necklace made of gold with a tiny heart locket hanging on the dainty chain. On the heart locket sat a beautiful little blue bird with its wings outstretched.

"That is to remind you that you are now free to be yourself girl. You will be safe here with us and we will treat you well. You can stay here for as long as you like and if you wish, never return to the orphanage. We paid for you not to work you hard, but to give you a new start."

Mrs. Noonan walked over to the girl who was staring at her in disbelief.

Above her bed, Shirley had noticed a framed picture of Jesus on the cross, and the kind lady now pointed to it and Shirley followed her finger to the picture.

"Just like the Lord Jesus Christ paid for our sins on the cross, so that we could be born again and set free."

Mrs. Noonan was obviously a good Catholic woman who lived the things she believed in. Shirley kept staring at the picture and then the necklace and then the picture again.

"We will talk about these things another time Shirley. Meanwhile though, I want to help you put your things away and then we will take a look around the house and garden."

The truly Christian woman opened drawers and unpacked the child's meagre possessions. She determined in her heart to find the wee lass some nice new things to cheer her up and to help demonstrate to the girl her worth. It was obvious to anyone who cared and was at all discerning that Shirley wore shame like a cape around her young shoulders. Mrs. Noonan sighed deeply, not wanting to think of the things that had given birth to this shame. Stretching up to her full height, wincing at the pain, she held her head high and walked to the door.

"Come along lass. Let's see if you like your new home. I have no doubt at all that we are going to like you very much indeed."

Chapter Thirty Four

"Forget injuries. Never forget kindnesses." Unknown

The Noonans had not been blessed with children and had adopted a girl they called Edie. She had grown into a "no-nonsense" girl and saw immediately that their little "acquisition" from the Catholic Orphanage was a "keeper." Edie was married to Bob and they both loved little Shirley. Whenever they were in Adelaide, they took her out with them to the pictures, the beach, on picnics, and to visit friends. They wanted to make up for all the things that they guessed she had missed out on. Shirley never talked about her life up until the day she came to live with "the Noonans."

Edith Ward was the Matron of the Pt. Pirie Hospital and her parents were rightfully proud of her. She was bright and she was kind and she was efficient. No matter what was happening in her life, Edie was always strong, down to earth, matter of fact and very respectful to her parents. She was their only child and all of their worldly goods were left to Edie in their wills.

This surprised Shirley, as she had not been exposed to adoption before and did not fully understand all that it meant. No-one had ever taught her that being adopted meant becoming part of the family as if the adoptee had actually been born into the family. She always felt that the Noonans were so kind to take Edie in and make her "like a daughter." The fact that she actually was their daughter escaped her. (In years to come, when some of her own grandchildren were also adopted, she still felt the same way.)

The young girl especially loved Saturday nights. They were quiet and peaceful and there was always the ritual of setting the table ready for Sunday lunch. This was a much-loved tradition in the household, and Sunday lunches were formal and delicious. Shirley blushed when Mr. Noonan teased her and she loved his twinkling eyes and sense of humour. He always seemed to find something to laugh about. He and Mrs. Noonan were very happy together and there was always a peaceful atmosphere in the house. Bob tried to outdo his father-in-law with joking around and on one occasion when they were all sitting at the table for Sunday lunch, Shirley dropped her serviette and had to bend down to retrieve it. Bob chirped up

"Oh my….and I thought she was shy! Shirley was just playing with my ankle!"

Everyone at the table fell about laughing and the object of their laughter turned the colour of beetroot. She loved the teasing though and knew that it was innocent. It was like being family. She told this story over and over again for the rest of her days.

She so loved her time with the Noonans that when Shirley had her first daughter, Edie became her Godmother and Mrs. Noonan became Godmother to her second. This was the best gift Shirley could give these two exceptional women.

After housing Shirley for three years, Thomas Noonan's health was failing. Nora Noonan's "Creeping Paralysis" was escalating. Her bike came in handy more and more. Edie talked with her parents and persuaded them it was time for Shirley to go out into the world and make her way. Edie assured her parents that her network with hospital staff would ensure a reliable live-in position for the young woman. Finally they gave in and broke the news to Shirley.

Someone to Watch Over Me

With mixed feelings the fourteen year old accepted her fate and braced her shoulders for yet another change in her young life.

"Carry your cross Shirley. You are a good, reliable, hard-working girl and you will do well out there in the world. I know it is hard for you to leave here, but you will find that working as a nurses' aid at the Ru Rua Hospital will be a very good job indeed. Edie has done a good thing in talking with Matron there, and singing your praises. You know - one matron to another."

Mrs. Noonan could not contain her pleasure as she spoke of the daughter of whom she was so proud.

"Your sleeping quarters are adequate and clean and you know how to do as you are told. Keep God's commandments and follow Him. It is the only way to live life and to be full of joy. Never forget, we Noonans will always be your family."

Shirley could hardly see the dear lady's face as her tears blurred her vision. The tremor in the kindly old voice indicated that her benefactor cared for her deeply and was also feeling sad at their parting.

Working around the house to assist Mrs. Noonan had been easy. Just like a daughter would do. There was a bit of dusting, especially of the treasured ornaments, and Shirley had been instructed right from the start about caution, slow movements, concentration and care. She had become accustomed to tidying up the house and doing some grocery shopping. She loved the walk along Prospect Road, with the basket over her arm and the occasional walk through St. Helen's Park.

Sometimes, sitting on the garden seat under the big tree, she would find herself chatting with some of the ladies as they watched their children play. One day it suddenly dawned on her that she no longer stuttered. With a grateful heart she realised that this too was something to thank Mrs. Noonan for. She had taught her well on many subjects.

Someone to Watch Over Me

Dear Mrs. Noonan had never doubted or judged her. She was a wise woman, straight-laced, and she had a heart of gold. Shirley had found a grand-mother in her and had found, through her family, that there were good, gentle, fair and loving men and women in the world.

The dreaded moment of farewell finally arrived. Shirley stopped her mind from meandering and focused on the moment. Her small suitcase was packed and sitting inside the screen door as if it was ready to go. She took a last, lingering look around the living room which she had painstakingly dusted and swept many times. So many memories.......a priest, a sponge cake with mock raspberry jam and vanilla custard filling. A scared and broken little girl with shameful secrets. Her mind was wandering again. Mrs. Noonan was sitting in her favourite chair, watching her and trying to smile. Overwhelmed with gratitude, she ran to her and flung herself against her huge bosom. They both let the dam burst. They had spent a great deal of time together over the last three years and a deep love and respect had been the result. The young girl had become a young woman and in the process had found a mother and grandmother wrapped in the same package.

Finally Shirley pulled herself away and thanked her kind friend for everything she could think of. Mrs. Noonan wiped her eyes on a lace handkerchief and spoke with difficulty.

"My precious child, it has been a blessing from God to have you in our home. May He go with you and keep you safe and guide you throughout your life. I will be praying for you and always remembering you in my heart."

Unable to speak, Shirley nodded her head and smiled her response. Slowly she pulled herself away and walked to the door, picking up her case, she opened the screen door for the last time and walked from her home and family. The family that the Lord Jesus Christ had given her. He had answered her prayers, eventually. Walking through the garden, she opened the gate and then closed it behind her, a metaphor for what was happening as

Someone to Watch Over Me

the door closed on this part of her life. She set off for Prospect Road, where she would catch a tram to Ru Rua Hospital to her new job and living quarters and hopefully, new friends.

Chapter Thirty Five

*"My grace is enough; it's all you need.
My strength comes into its own in your weakness."*
2 Corinthians 12:9 The Message

Her room was clean and bare.

It was not like her beautiful room that she had just left behind.

There was a small wardrobe for her belongings.

There was a single bed, no dressing table, cupboard or shelf.

She would make do.

The telephone in the sleep-out was for all the girls to share. They were allowed to use it in their own time. A much appreciated luxury. A way to keep in touch at last.

The work was as she expected, very demanding. Easy though, when comparison was made with the slave labour at the orphanage and on the Carrieton property. Even the bedpans were not too bad, so long as she held her breath when she emptied them, and tried not to look at the contents. She had a uniform and looked like a real nurse. She looked pretty and when there were any boys around, they would give her an interested second glance. No-one seemed to notice her blind eye, and she certainly wasn't going to mention it. Her good eye worked really well, and seemed to make up adequately for her other one. What else could she ask for? She had a bed, food and a small income. She also had fun and chats with the other maids and the beginnings of friendship.

Some days she would walk with her new friend Gwen Button and watch the Piccadilly Theatre being constructed. They could not wait for it to be finished so that they could go together and see some of the romantic musicals that were the current craze.

Once a week, Shirley allowed herself a ritual that brought her much pleasure. She would travel by tram into the city to Balfour's Cafeteria and treat herself to a cherry tart and a cup of tea. She felt like she was a real lady and even a "bit of a toff." These outings were precious attempts at normality because she had no family to catch up with on days off. Visiting Balfour's became her familiar place to go and the familiar staff her well-known faces.

Sadly, Shirley became ill quite suddenly and could not go to work for a few days or to Balfour's. It was difficult for her to even lift her head from the pillow. The other nurses' maids became very concerned for her, especially as her weight plummeted rapidly. A doctor was called in from one of the wards and he diagnosed pneumonia. Shirley was kept on the balcony at Ru Rua Hospital overnight and then transferred to the Royal Adelaide Hospital the next day. She was kept on the balcony there as well. It was similar to a sleep-out and was used for patients when the rest of the hospital was full. There was an old canvas water bag hanging nearby providing drinks for the patients.

Shirley had her glass filled from this regularly as her fever made her very thirsty. She could not face food and it took her some time to recover and regain her strength and appetite. Her friend Gwen came to see her and broke the sad news that she had been replaced at Ru Rua. Shirley stared at the ceiling over her bed and cried.

"Where will I live? How will I survive with no money? Where will I get a live- in job? What will happen to me? I have no-one to take care of me."

Someone to Watch Over Me

Her friend went to her and held her as the lonely girl realised she was destitute with no back-up.

Pulling herself together, the teen-ager told herself that she would work things out on her own, and that something would come up. Her strong fighting spirit, developed during the many hardships in her young life, enabled her to determine that she would not give up but keep on fighting. She said goodbye to Gwen and then lay on her hospital bed, weakened and ill, but not beaten.

While she was still recuperating on the balcony of the Royal Adelaide Hospital, she had two more visitors. They cheered her up no end. Somehow they had heard about her illness and had managed to trace her. They were sisters, almost her sisters, because they were from St. Joseph's Orphanage. Muriel and Anna had found her. They brought food. Temptations she could not easily resist, because they had purchased the treat with their own hard-earned money. Sitting in a white cardboard box were six adorable, very green frog cakes. Balfour's specialty. A huge treat for any sweet-tooth. Shirley stared at the green frogs as they smiled their wide creamy smile at her and she cried.

"If we thought you'd be disappointed, we'd have bought finger buns," Muriel joked.

The three friends burst into giggles.

"Let's have a party!" exclaimed Anna and they all nodded, tucking into the delicacies.

The unexpected visit from her two old friends was a turning point in her recovery and after a few days Shirley was up and dressed and asking around about possible live-in positions. She had been saved by love - and frog cakes.

One of her fellow patients told her about a possible opening on Prospect Road. A wealthy family were looking for a live-in maid. Their name was Lawrence and they owned a very successful business in the city. The eager girl quickly looked up the number in the directory which sat next to a public telephone

Someone to Watch Over Me

in the hospital. She was relieved to find a few pennies in her purse, and she dropped the right amount into the slot and dialled the number. As she dialled, she crossed herself as she had learned in the orphanage and then prayed to Mary and Jesus, Father God, the Holy Spirit and also any Saint who was listening to help her get this live-in job.

When the person at the other end of the line said they would like to meet her and named a time that afternoon, she almost fainted. Excitedly checking in her purse again, and hoping for a miracle, she worked out that she could follow the instructions and travel by tram some of the distance and then walk the rest of the way to Audley House, which was situated on Prospect Road. Realising that she was very weak from her illness, the determined young lady also realised that desperation would make up for that and she just had to get this position. There was no-one to ask for a lift, and no money for a taxi, so a tram-car ride some of the way would do, and a walk all the way back to the hospital afterwards was something to worry about later on.

Quickly running a comb through her hair, she smoothed her crumpled dress down with her hands, One of her fellow patients loaned her a pair of stockings and a hat and she thanked her warmly as she hurried out of the door, her heart racing with anxiety and hope.

After a very long walk for the right tram, she was exhausted. The tram ride along Prospect Road would be short because she did not have the right fare. She would need to walk the rest of the distance. She explained to the conductor and asked him to tell her when to get off because her fare had run out.

Upon quizzing her further and discovering that she was on her way to an interview for a live-in position, the conductor turned a blind eye and offered to let her know when they arrived at Audley House. Pulling the cord to ring the bell to alert the driver, the conductor smiled at her.

Someone to Watch Over Me

"Here you are lassie. That's Audley House over there. The side street's been named after it. Some rich folk must live in there I reckon. I hear they are good people. Good luck to ya."

With a smile she thanked him and gave him a friendly wave as the tram took off again along Prospect Road. Standing at the gate to the grand house, fear grabbed at her knees and she froze. It enveloped her, bringing with it a sense of unworthiness and shame and shattering any confidence that she had in her abilities. Shaking her head she fought off her demons and walked steadily up the garden path to the front door.

She rang the doorbell.

The door was opened.

She forgot to say hello and to introduce herself. All she could do was apologise. She was worried that she might be judged unfairly and lose this incredible opportunity.

"I am so sorry that I am late. I had to come a long way, from the city, and I didn't have enough money for the journey, so I had to walk a very long way, and then wait for the right tram. I didn't have a time table. I didn't have a map and had to ask a few times for directions, and the nice tram conductor let me stay on the tram, even though I didn't have the right money, and I always try to be on time, but I couldn't help it."

She stopped her furtive explanations when she saw the smile on the face of the man at the door.

"It's all right Shirley. I take it that you are Shirley who rang me earlier today?"

"Yes. I am."

"You showed me many great character traits just then, and I am impressed. Your determination and ability to rise to the occasion, in spite of the hurdles in your way, your concern for punctuality, your good manners in apologising for being late, even though it was unavoidable. All these things show me that we are going to get along very well indeed."

Her fear was dispelled. He was not going to hold anything against her. He seemed to like her and to be a fair man.

Tears welled in her eyes and spilled over, running down her cheeks.

"How kind of you. Thank you."

"Come on inside lass and let's have a cup of tea and a chat. I'm sure we can work something out and I will drive you back to where you need to go afterwards. It sounds like your purse has run out of pennies."

Mr. Lawrence was a good judge of character and he sensed that this young lady had suffered a great deal. Her loneliness was easy to read and the fact that she was unsupported and needing a live-in job at such a young age moved him. He was a charitable soul and was not opposed to using the power that he had as a successful businessman to turn around a life when given the opportunity. His business, "Lawrence the Tobacconist" was located on the iconic Bee-Hive Corner where Rundle Mall and King William Street joined in Adelaide City.

He ushered her into the kitchen and asked the cook to rustle up some refreshments. They settled themselves at the table to chat. Upon hearing that she had come straight from hospital, where she was a recovering patient from pneumonia, he reassured her that he would like to give her the position, and she could come straight to Audley House once she was discharged. Her eyes welled with tears of relief and gratitude. Fishing in his breast pocket, he drew out a handkerchief for her, and then his trouser pocket gave up a handful of coins, which he pressed into her hand.

"This should get you back here to us once you are discharged lassie. Now, if you've finished your tea and biscuit, I'll show you around and I'm sure you'd like to see your room as well. You might like to know that we will provide a uniform for you too and pay you a small wage. The rest of your pay covers your accommodation, including all meals, which I think you'll enjoy. Our cook is one of the best."

The cook turned around from the stove where she was stirring something in a large saucepan and smiled at the compliment giver. Mr. Lawrence winked at Shirley and the sense of belonging and camaraderie swept into her heart.

When she stood to her feet, relief and joy and gratitude all tumbled around in her head, making her feel giddy momentarily. It passed and she couldn't help smiling. She felt like singing, but thought that had better wait for a more appropriate time.

Thank you Heavenly Father. You keep on helping me, when all seems hopeless and lost. I don't deserve it. But Mrs. Noonan said you love everyone. I guess you must love me too, just like she said. You keep putting good people there for me. Mrs. Noonan said she would keep praying for me. Everything has changed since she came into my life.

She felt for her bluebird necklace and remembered the words of her benefactor and friend.

Jesus died for me, just like He died for everyone. I am included. I'm not left out in the cold.

Chapter Thirty Six

"The service we render to others is really the rent we pay for our room on this earth." Wilfred Grenfell

What a relief! What an enormous relief!
The words kept racing through her head, over and over again. She had somewhere to live, food to eat, an income to save from, and nice people to work for. A roof over her head. A bed to sleep in. All this in perfect timing. All thanks to someone speaking up and helping her in the hospital. Sitting on her bed in her new room she fidgeted with her tram ticket, grateful for that provision as well. It was like someone was watching over her and taking care of her, even though she couldn't see them.

She folded and unfolded the ticket as she thought of what might have been, if things did not go as they had for her. *I must try to be there for others like that. What a difference it has made to me when people are kind.*

Looking around her room she contemplated how it was positioned at the back of the large mansion, away from the main living area. It hit her that it was very quiet in her room. She remembered the hustle and bustle and noise of the nurses' quarters. Everyone seemed to talk at once, complaining about nurses, doctors, patients and mess to clean up. Then there would be talk about favourite patients or handsome doctors or interns. There was constant activity and sharing of possessions and hints and opinions. There were broken nails and broken hearts. A new pretty dress someone wanted to show off. Or a new boyfriend to brag about. The one 'phone they shared was always occupied and this link to the outside world was a constant source of news and gossip. It felt like she belonged to a community. Would things go well here? Would she have friends? Would something turn up to fill the emptiness?

Shaking off the melancholy, like a wet puppy shaking off rain drops, she looked around her room. There was a dressing table, a single bed with a wire base and a comfy looking mattress. The sheets were a pale blue and a pretty feather eiderdown in pastel shades sat on top. The wardrobe was a one door piece of furniture, but more than adequate for her one dress, one blouse, one pair of black trousers and her much loved navy overcoat, given to her by her friend Anna. She would like to buy a hat one day when she saved enough to go shopping. This imagined hat would perch sweetly on top of the wardrobe in a hat box, she decided. In the bottom of the wardrobe were two folded spare blankets and another pillow. To her delight, hanging inside was a maid's uniform in black, with a frilly white apron and the cutest little lacy head-dress she had ever seen. Quickly, Shirley wriggled into the uniform. She stood staring at herself in the mirror and smiled and curtsied to the pretty little French maid who curtsied while smiling back at her. The little lacy hairpiece sat amongst her curls and she knew she looked a picture.

I wish the girls at Ru Rua could see me now. Mrs. Noonan would be impressed, too. I'll have to tell her all about this place when I get to visit her. And my father would be proud if he knew. I'm sure he would.

Quickly she brushed away the thoughts of her father and polished her shoes. She found her stockings in the bottom of her case and put them on, then her shoes and critically checked out the result. Speaking in a deep voice, she pretended to be Mr. Lawrence.

"Well my dear, you'll have to do because there's no-one else here to dust and clean."

Someone to Watch Over Me

Laughing at herself she tidied up her room, checked the time on her watch, and decided it was time to emerge from her room and see what work was waiting for her.

The house was massive. There were many rooms upstairs and downstairs. The polished floors made her scowl.

My poor housewife's knees, she thought to herself.

There were several bathrooms, and two lounge rooms. She knew that she would get very fit looking after this house. Each day she dusted, cleaned and tidied, swept, polished, scrubbed and mopped and then collapsed at the end of the day and slept like a baby. In between times she hungrily devoured her meals, needing to replenish the energy just spent. Very soon she was in a routine with her chores, which included laying and clearing tables, washing dishes and assisting the cook whenever she required help.

During the meal times, Shirley waited on the table and was taught to always serve from the left of the person and remove the plates from the right. Sometimes she slipped up and went from the wrong side. This seemed to amuse Mr. Lawrence considerably when the anxious girl became embarrassed, blushed deeply and then fumbled around trying to correct her mistake, all the time whispering her apologies, as if she had committed the unpardonable sin.

The Lawrences loved to entertain and they especially loved to have people over to play Bridge. Shirley wore her uniform at all times and served eats and drinks to the table, for the guests. She was proud of her tiny waist and knew that her legs were "not too bad" because the girls at Ru Rua had told her so. This knowledge bolstered her self confidence a little as she stood near the Bridge table, constantly at the ready for guests' requests. She blushed when she was noticed and spoken to directly. It amazed her that the guests seemed to like her and that it amused them to tease her. Sometimes they asked her questions about her life and were intrigued with the pretty little maid who was completely alone in the world.

Shirley remained secretive about her background until one evening a jolly gentleman dressed in a pin-striped suit and shiny red tie asked for her surname.

"Shirley who?" he enquired.

The other guests at the table stopped what they were doing and looked in her direction. The quietness was palpable as they awaited her reply. It would have been rude to ignore him and she couldn't think fast enough to make up a name so she blurted out the truth.

"Shirley Gilfillan, Sir."

"Gilfillan eh? Well that's not a name you come across a lot Shirley. Would your father's Christian name be Percy, by any chance?"

The young girl was pouring beer into a glass at the time, and she lost control and some splashed all over the table.

"Are you alright little one? You look as if you have just seen a ghost."

The jolly gentleman looked concerned.

"Would you like to sit down?"

Someone was asking her something and handing her a drink of water all at the same time.

A chair was drawn up and she was helped into it. One of the kindly ladies in a beautiful dark blue dress fanned her with her prettily hand painted fan. Everything was blurred and in slow motion and she found it hard to concentrate. The haziness and drumming in her head warned Shirley that she was about to faint. Someone told her to take deep breaths. She obeyed them and gradually felt better.

The jolly gentleman approached her again, but this time more gingerly.

"I take it from your reaction, Shirley, that your father's name is Percy. Is he a french polisher?"

Shirley nodded.

"I know him," said the jolly gentleman. "He works in the city, in Savery's. I was just talking with him the other day. He seems like a fine, responsible man. I am sure that he would want to hear from you."

Well, that would be the first time in years, if he did, thought the girl, but she did not speak it out.

"You should telephone him and set up a time to meet. I am sure that he would be very proud of you indeed. You are such a lovely young lass, and you have a good job with live-in keep in this beautiful mansion and for these successful, and well-known and much-liked business people."

The man was now trying to impress his hosts. He was keen to stay on their invitation list for their Bridge parties.

"All right then, I will try to telephone him during the week, if this is alright with Mr. and Mrs. Lawrence."

Shirley was embarrassed at the huge amount of interest in her and her story. All eyes around the table were on her and she quickly pushed back her chair and resumed her position as maid, instead of the heroine in some romantic novel.

"Of course Shirley, you can ring tomorrow morning if you wish. Then you can tell us all at our next Bridge meeting just how it went with you and your father."

Mrs. Lawrence was obviously intrigued, like everyone else around the table.

The maid nodded her gratitude and stepped back from the table, retreating to the kitchen to catch her breath. She knew that catching up with her father, assuming he wanted to catch up with her at all, meant hearing news about her mother. The young lass was not sure if she wanted this door opened to her and she certainly did not want anyone to know about her poor mother living out her days in a mental institution. Shrugging her shoulders and patting her hair, feeling to see if her lacy little

Someone to Watch Over Me

head-dress was still there, she busied herself helping the cook with the washing up and other kitchen duties.

Without a word, but with a definite compassionate look, 'Cook' had placed a very welcome hot cup of sweetened tea before her and kindly patted her on her shoulder. Shirley explained that she did not want to go back into the dining room tonight and 'Cook' nodded her understanding and took over Shirley's duties whilst the girl looked after the kitchen. The cook seemed to understand that her young charge had had enough excitement and attention for one night.

Tomorrow she would telephone her father and find out if he was willing to meet her. Would he want to see her, when he had made no move to do so in all these years? Where should she suggest for their meeting? What should she wear? If she looked her very best, perhaps he would be impressed and want to see his daughter again. Maybe he had other children? Would she get to meet them?

It was not too big a choice as Shirley owned only a few pieces of clothing and one change of underwear. The decision was made quickly. She would wear her blue dress and buy a pretty little hat to go with it. She would try to meet him after work on a Thursday night on North Terrace. She would choose a particular seat and sit there, waiting for him like the grown up she now was. He would have to like her. The jolly gentleman said so.

The morning finally came, after a sleepless night of tossing and turning. She faced the telephone in the hallway and wiped her hands, sweaty with anxiety. There was a lump in her throat that she tried to clear with a little cough. Her throat felt tight and when she went to speak, only a squeak came out.

I sound like a mouse, she thought to herself with a nervous laugh. She practised speaking again, as she dialled the number for Savery's.

"May I speak with Percy Gilfillan please. He is a french polisher."

Someone to Watch Over Me

This was spoken with a touch of pride.

She waited and almost gave up, when someone picked up the telephone.

"Hello."

"Are you Percy Gilfillan?" *That was better*, she thought, even though it was only a whisper.

"Yes, I am Percy Gilfillan."

His voice was pleasant.

"I am Shirley."

Silence.

"Shirley Gilfillan."

He still did not speak.

"I was told that you worked at Saverys."

She was scared that he would hang up on her and she desperately wanted to meet him.

Finally he spoke. Now his voice seemed to be a whisper too.

"I always knew you would find me someday."

"I would like to meet you sometime."

Her words were quick this time as she was anxious to arrange a meeting.

"Yes. Of course. But not at my work. Do you work, Shirley, or are you at school?"

She understood that he did not want his workmates to know about her. A pain seemed to grab her in her chest. He was ashamed of her.

Then he spoke again.

"What I mean is when would it suit you to meet me?"

The young woman was glad that she had formed a plan before making her phone call. She quickly mentioned the seat on North Terrace and Percy suggested a time, one week ahead, after he knocked off from work. The arrangement was made. They said their goodbyes. The fifteen year old fell into the kitchen chair as Mrs. Lawrence watched on with concern and interest.

"It is arranged. He wants to meet me."

Someone to Watch Over Me

There were no more words because the girl suddenly burst into a fit of bottled up sobs. With her face in her hands, her shoulders shook. Deep longings rose to the surface at last, as they were given permission to appear from hiding. Her daddy. At last. She had a family. She was not an orphan.

The anxious girl stood frozen to the spot as she glared at the china cup that she had just dropped. Its pretty pattern of roses was now scattered into many pieces on the polished floor. Mrs. Lawrence was frowning at her and she knew she was in trouble.

"I am truly sorry," whispered the worried lass.

Her employer quickly read Shirley's remorse and knew that chastisement was not necessary in this case.

Shirley had dropped two other pieces of china in as many days. She was a nervous wreck awaiting the meeting with her father.

"Shirley, I just want to know if I will have any china left in one piece by the time you finally meet this father of yours?"

Their eyes met, and the two women exchanged smiles.

She hurried into the library and dusted frantically. Two days to go. She tried to concentrate on removing the dust from the bookshelves. The goal was to distract herself, but the mounting excitement blocked out whatever she was doing. All she could think of was herself sitting on the bench seat wearing her old blue dress and pretty little brand new blue felt hat with the ice pink rose on the side.

Chapter Thirty Seven

"The time is always right to do what is right." Martin Luther King Jnr.

He isn't coming, she thought.

She had been sitting in the one position, for ages, posed prettily with a smile which had faded like a summer rose. Her tiny gold wrist-watch that kindly Mrs. Lawrence had given to her from her collection of watches proclaimed that it was actually fifteen minutes past their meeting time.

He must have forgotten. He doesn't want to face me. His guilt over abandoning me won out. He is too busy. He doesn't want to be reminded of those bad days with his crazy wife. He thinks I might be like her. He is worried I will want money from him.....and he hasn't paid a half-penny to help me in all these years. I want nothing from him. The b........, she thought when suddenly, the silence was broken.

"Hello Shirley."

She was frozen in a huge block of ice. She could not breathe. She did not respond.

"I'm sorry that I'm late. The boss needed to talk with me about a special customer's requirements and I couldn't get away. I hope you didn't think I had stood you up."

He is being his most charming, she thought to herself. She noticed that he looked a little uncomfortable, avoiding her eyes with his. She tried to remember what he looked like when she saw him, so many years ago. Years without a glimpse of him - or even a photograph to remind her of her father. She had a vague memory of black, slick hair. Now it was peppered with grey and dull and thinning. He was of average height, although he had seemed very tall when she was a child. He looked impressive, nevertheless, in his dark suit, white shirt and navy striped tie. She guessed that he had dressed to impress her, not usually turning up to do his french polishing in a suit.

He stared at her. She stared back.

Shirley still had not spoken and the words just would not come. She looked at her hands and noticed that they were trembling. She didn't want him to see that she was anxious.

"I am so glad to see you all grown up. I've wanted to get in touch with you, but always seemed to be busy...." His voice trailed off as he heard his own hurtful, abandoning and feeble words of explanation.

He fiddled with his hat, which he held in both of his hands.

"Here, I thought you might like to meet someone. Come here Molly. This is Shirley...my....eh...girl.. you know, I told you about her."

A short, dumpy, sour looking woman stepped towards them. Shirley had not realised that she was with him until this moment. She disliked her immediately. She did not understand what their relationship was, but could not believe that he would bring his woman friend to this reunion with his long lost daughter. She felt jealousy for her poor mother, who was still married to her father. She had found this out recently.

Shirley wanted her father to herself, especially right now, as they were meeting for the first time in so many lonely years. Nasty black emotions rose from the depths of her soul and fought inside her. Anger, fury, resentment, bitterness, hurt and despair.

When would my father ever get it? Would he ever understand how I have longed for him and pleaded with God to remind him that he had a daughter? Year after year. Watching for him. Waiting and waiting. Not even a birthday card or

Someone to Watch Over Me

something at Christmas. Forgotten. For years. Then he brings his lady friend and thinks I might like to meet her? Would he like to know what I would like to do to this nasty woman who keeps glaring at me? This woman who is looking me up and down critically. This woman who has had your attention when I have had your rejection. Better keep her out of my sight or I might give her more than she bargains for. Shirley had many words cascading through her mind at a rapid rate, but she still had not spoken.

The awareness of the importance of this moment in her life hit her like lightening and she chastised herself. Nodding towards Molly she managed to speak in a whisper.

"Hello," was the best she could do.

Her father relaxed a little as the tension was broken with one word. He asked his daughter about her employment and accommodation and was impressed to hear about the jolly gentleman and his clue to where her father worked. The trio of strangers laughed together at her story of spilling the beer all over the bridge table when she was told about her father. She was relieved to sense her heart thawing and surprised at how much better it felt when she laughed. Not knowing what to call her father she settled with calling him nothing for the time being.

Struggling to bring her mind back to this critical moment in time, the young lady heard her father inviting her to a meal at his place, and suggesting that he would pick her up from Audley House late on Saturday afternoon in his old Dodge, then drive her back later that night. The plan was agreed upon and then they all awkwardly said goodbye. Shirley set out to catch her tram back to Audley House. Sitting on the tram she thought about the encounter and decided that it went better than expected. She had wanted to scream at him and beat his chest with her clenched fists. Hurt him for all the hurt he had caused her.

Somehow she had behaved well and kept control and her prize was an invitation to their home. She had longed to have him hug her and apologise and assure her of his affection, but maybe that would come down the track. Telling herself to be thankful for this triumph and shrugging her shoulders, the feisty young lass promised that the bottled-up words would be said when the time was right.

Chapter Thirty Eight

"Those who bring sunshine into the lives of others cannot keep it from themselves." James M. Barrie

The fifteen year old had been at the Lawrence's for almost a year now and her relationship with her father had settled into regular visits. Mostly their time together was pleasant, but Shirley was aware that Molly was jealous of any affection that Percy bestowed upon his daughter. Percy was aware, also, and he felt pushed and pulled between the two women.

When it was time for him to drive his daughter home, each Saturday, Molly would insist on coming along, even if the dishes and cleaning up were unfinished. She would quickly position herself into the front seat alongside the driver, leaving Shirley to the window seat, and separated from her father. Molly would control the talking, choosing subjects that Shirley was unfamiliar with, therefore forcing her out of the conversation.

At one stage Percy had bought Shirley a small gift and Molly had made sarcastic comments, suggesting that she was looking forward to her gift next time. The air was heavy and Molly always managed to take the shine off any special moments between Percy and his only child.

Noticing how many people rode bikes around the streets, Shirley happened to remark one evening how she would dearly love to have a bike. She went on to say that she had never learned to ride one and that her idea was probably foolish.

Her father reminded her of this conversation when they eventually had some time alone. Molly had a headache and could not face the trip to accompany Shirley back to Audley House. Shirley and Percy travelled together, chatting freely, as he drove her back to her place of employment.

"Shirl, me girl. Do you still want to learn to ride a bike?"

"Of course. I just don't know how it's ever going to happen."

"Well, your luck has changed. I am going to teach you."

He looked very pleased with himself.

"How are you going to manage that Dad? I can't see Molly letting you spend that sort of time with me."

She resented the older woman's power over her father.

"Well, love, it will have to be our secret. But I have managed to get hold of a bike for you, and my neighbour, you know Syd Jeffrey, well, he is going to keep it in his shed. We'll have to go there first of all when you come for a visit, so I'll pick you up an hour early each time. We'll park the Dodge around the corner and Molly will never know the difference."

He was chuckling and gave her a cheeky wink.

"However will you explain leaving early to pick me up but getting back late?"

Knowing Molly's retribution tactics, Shirley did not want to be in the firing line again, should the older woman discover their secret.

"I'll just tell her that I've decided to call into the pub for a few beers with the boys, and to place a few bets on the gee-gees. She won't give it two thoughts."

Shirley finally allowed herself excitement about their plan. It would be good to put one over on the 'evil Molly', for sure. It was a thrill to share a secret with her father. Their first conspiracy. Soon she would have her own means of transport. Thanks to her dad. Life was looking up.

Chapter Thirty Nine

"Change always comes bearing gifts." Price Pritchett

There was tension in the house. Whispers were shared. Staff were given notice. Shirley had only a week to find a new live-in position. She was sixteen and homeless. Once again the fear grabbed at her heart like bony fingers, squeezing tightly. She took deep breaths and assured herself that something would turn up. It always did. She prayed, calling out to her Heavenly Father to rescue her.

She spoke to her earthly father and asked for his help, too. Shirley hoped that he would take her into his home with Molly and her mother. He was only a boarder there, in their rented house, so had no say and her hopes were quickly dashed.

The days flashed past with no light on the horizon. Desperation started to set in and Shirley considered begging Molly to take her in until something turned up.

On her second to last day at the stately Audley House, the stressed-out lass heard of a position for a live-in house-maid in Prospect with the Brogans. It was also on Prospect Road, a short distance north of her current home. She quickly rang the lady of the house, mentioning her previous live-in positions, and secured an appointment for later in the day, when she finished work.

Standing on Prospect Road, her bike leaning against the fence, she placed her hand on the latch of the large gate. Shirley was in awe as she gazed up at the pretty-as-a-picture bull-nosed veranda house with two tall chimneys reaching up to the sky, with spectacular stone work, an enchanting roof with a variety of roof angles and a decorative iron treatment around the two large verandas. It was a grand, intimidating yet beautiful house. Almost a dozen steps led up to the villa, with pillars standing like sentinels on either side. The front door had colourful lead-light on each side and the many posts to the veranda were hand-turned timber and pretty to look at. The decorative iron-pressed trim was repeated at the bottom of the posts, joining them with a fence-like arrangement.

Opening the gate, Shirley walked through and up the steps to the front door. She had noticed another door around the side of the house, which also looked like an entrance, and she was confused. *Which door am I supposed to knock on?* Shaking off her confusion, she decided to knock on the main entrance door and with hope in her heart, she did so while praying for courage.

Please dear Lord, may this be my new home. Let them like me. Let me say the right thing.

The door was opened by a friendly looking woman in her early fifties. She smiled warmly at Shirley, seeming to like what she saw right from the first moment. The younger woman relaxed right away and took a deep breath.

"Shirley, I have spoken with Mrs. Noonan, and Mrs. Lawrence, your two previous employers, and you have been given great references. We will have a cup of tea together and get to know each other. I suspect you will fit in here very well indeed. Mr. Brogan will be along shortly so you can meet him as well. We are in a dreadful mess right now because we are doing some decorating and there are three painters here and drop sheets, ladders and scaffolding, brushes and paint tins all over the place. It is going to look amazing, but we will all have to be tolerant and patient right now."

Shirley smiled back and nodded her head as the lady of the house showed her into the kitchen.

Someone to Watch Over Me

"Take a seat at the table dear girl and I will put the kettle on. If you decide you like it here, we will not work you hard but you will become part of the family. Now how do you take your tea?"

The two women chatted and enjoyed their tea with home-made cockle biscuits, joined with raspberry jam with a pink icing on top which was sprinkled with coconut.

Shirley could hear the three painters whistling and talking somewhere nearby in one of the rooms and thought it a warm background to her conversation with the friendly Mrs. Brogan. She decided that this would be a perfect place to live-in and serve in and she liked Mrs. Brogan from the first moment when she opened the door with a smile and a warm welcome.

It was decided. Shirley would move in at the end of her final day at Audley House tomorrow. Her room sounded adequate, and had already been re-painted. Mrs. Brogan led her to it so that she would know what to expect and she was delighted to see that it was adjacent to the bathroom and toilet.

Picking up her handbag, Shirley decided that she should take her leave and thank Mrs. Brogan graciously for accepting her. As the two women were saying their good-byes, a well dressed gentleman came into the hallway, having entered the house from the side door entrance.

"Well, what do we have here? Is this the young woman that you mentioned to me, Mrs. Brogan?"

"Let me introduce you to our new live-in maid, Mr. Brogan. Meet Shirley Gilfillan, who will finish at Audley House tomorrow. What perfect timing don't you think? I have no doubt in my mind that she will fit in here very well indeed. She is a delightful, although secretive young lady. I could not get too much information from her about her history, but Mrs. Noonan and Mrs. Lawrence have told me all I need to know. We are very lucky to have her and I hope she will be happy here."

Someone to Watch Over Me

Mr. Brogan smiled a warm welcome and they chatted for a couple of minutes before Shirley excused herself and headed back on her bike to her home for one more night and day.

Pushing briskly on the pedals, she felt alive and excited enough to burst into song. So she did. Singing from her heart as she rode along Prospect Road, she sang out loud, *"Happy Days are Here Again,"*[3] remembering the movie that the nuns at St. Jo's had played several times on their old projector, on to the wall of the common room. She thought it was called *'Chasing Rainbows.'*

"That's me for sure. Always chasing rainbows and hoping that there will be a pot of gold at the bottom of one."

Little did she know that her pot of gold was about to be found.

---

[3] Composer Milton Ager, Lyrics by Jack Yellen

Chapter Forty

"We need to be at peace with our past, content with our present, and sure about our future, knowing they are all in God's hands."
Joyce Meyer

As quick as a flash, Shirley said her goodbyes, from a grateful heart to those at Audley House, picked up her small case, strapped it to her bike carriage and took off up the driveway, through the large gateway and onto Prospect Road. She settled in quickly, feeling very much at home with the Brogans and loving her newly painted room. A bright and sun shiny yellow, to match the hope in her heart. Very quickly Shirley adjusted to her new surroundings and worked very hard at her list of chores. When they were completed, her reward was to go out. She loved to do this and especially loved going to the picture theatre to see new movies.

The dance hall was a new passion that had entered her life and she saved every penny she could in order to catch the tram to "The Embassy" in Grenfell Street in the city. It had been love at first sight when her eyes fell on the swirling skirts of shiny and delicate fabrics in breath-taking colours that turned their wearers into film star impersonators. The combination of toe-tapping music, ruffles, gathers, pleats and frills mesmerised the lass as she sat on her chair against the wall, wishing to be one of the magnificent dancers that were a picture of loveliness before her. Transported into a dream of a handsome prince escorting her to the dance floor and turning her into a princess, she knew this could never happen in reality. Looking down at her sad little dress and shabby shoes which had known better days, she felt more like a modern day Cinderella, without a fairy godmother, realising she was no competition at all for the ladies twirling in their splendid finery.

A young man stood in front of her and had been speaking so quietly and nervously, she had not heard him. His face was covered with blazing acne and his greasy hair hung over his pale blue eyes. What the band lacked in skill they made up for in enthusiasm, and they were beating out the newly-released popular song, *'I don't want to set the world on fire.'*[4]

Just as well. You'd have no chance, thought Shirley as she looked at the sorry-looking teenager who was eagerly awaiting her answer.

"Would you like to dance?"

The words were almost inaudible. He cleared his croaky throat and tried yet again.

Shirley knew what it was like to be rejected and could not hurt him. She rose to her feet and nodded. He offered the crook of his arm to her and she threaded her arm through, as he escorted her on to the parquetry floor. The dance floor was packed, so her self-consciousness at not knowing how to dance soon subsided as they melded into the crowd. As they danced awkwardly around and around the floor, the sixteen year-old found herself looking over her partner's shoulder, instead of at her poor trodden-on feet. She watched the other dancers and quickly picked up the steps. She had a great sense of rhythm and was pleased with herself at how well she was doing.

Suddenly Shirley was staring at one couple in particular, turning around again and again to keep her eyes on them. Her young partner noticed that she was gaping and looking longingly at someone, and he danced her around so that he could see who

---

[4] Released in 1941 by The Ink Spots

she was staring at. He noticed that she was smitten. When he saw the object of her attention, he sighed, and he thought he should have known without looking. The very handsome and extremely popular Burt was dancing, as usual, like a film star. Everyone called him Clark because he was thought to look like the star of the silver screen, Clark Gable. It was obvious that Burt agreed with them. Poor Joey also noticed that the dancers on the floor had cleared a space for Burt to shine as he 'tripped the light fantastic' with his usual dance partner Ida. Everyone seemed to be staring at the pair as they danced magnificently together.

Joey cleared his throat again and Shirley quickly came out of her trance, endeavouring to focus on dancing with Joey. They did not set the world on fire, but nevertheless they muddled their way through the number, without tripping themselves or anyone else up on the dance floor.

The young lady, in the sad little blue dress had several dances that night, but the only man she had eyes for was Burt. While sitting out dances, she watched him as he glided, non-stop, with his talented partner. They were amazing together and Shirley found herself day-dreaming about being that partner herself. A plan started to form in her active young mind. It involved a beautiful new dress and some dance lessons, and then?..... She wrestled over the next part of the plan. How would she ever get to steal him away from that woman who danced like the famous Ginger Rogers?

Tomorrow she would talk with Mrs. Brogan and get her advice. A woman like Mrs. Brogan would know what to do.

Chapter Forty One

"Dancing with the feet is one thing, but dancing with the heart is another." Anonymous

She looked beautiful. Not just nice, but stunning. The mirror said so. Her dress was fit for a princess, in icy pink and the dreamy fabric of organza. The gown had been cut perfectly into her tiny waist, and it flared out into a magnificent skirt with pretty ruffles. It was finished, in just one week, and it was perfect. As she stood and stared at her reflection, she forgot to breathe, momentarily. She was spellbound.

Mrs. Brogan had worked a miracle. She had asked her own dressmaker, Mrs. Renfrey, to put her other work aside and fast-track an urgent dress as a special favour for her best customer. Shirley had two fittings and had to try hard to remain still as the excitement caused her to be very animated.

"Save your energy for the dance-floor my girl. We want this young man to be gob-smacked when he lays eyes on you. If you want my opinion, he doesn't stand a chance. I have a feeling that you are going to need a big stick to fight off all those young men at the dance."

Mrs. Brogan was very proud of her achievement.

Shirley tried to remember to breathe. It wasn't that the dress was too tight. It was her amazement at seeing herself in such a lovely creation. The fabric looked like "gossamer wings" and the colour suited her beautifully. Joy filled her and she felt better than she ever had in her whole life. It was intoxicating, this joy. She looked normal. She looked lovely. Shirley the orphan. Shirley

Someone to Watch Over Me

the reject. Shirley the maid with no home. Now a princess. Whoever would have thought it possible. It was all too much and the wonderful feeling burst out into tears of bubbling happiness. A small seed of hope also burst into life in her heart.

Maybe he would notice her after all. She tenderly hung the princess dress in her wardrobe and longed for her next Saturday night off, so that she could go to The Embassy dance again. Mrs. Renfrey had given her a left-over piece of the dress fabric and she folded it carefully and then placed it under her pillow, hoping she would dream of herself and the handsome prince dancing together and everyone watching and marvelling at what a lovely couple they made.

She rose at 6:00 a.m. and put on her black with white trim maid's uniform, as usual, and after a quick breakfast she cleared up the dishes and headed for the front yard. She had been asked to weed the gravel driveway. The sun was shining and pleasantly warming on a fairly crisp morning. Exiting through the back door, she was careful to make her way around the paint tins, planks, drop sheets and buckets of brushes. She remembered that the painters were coming back to sand back the outside woodwork today, ready for a fresh new look to the house. Until now, she had only heard them as they painted the front rooms of the house. When they disappeared she was told that they had to go to another urgent job, but would be back in a couple of weeks to paint the outside of the Brogans' lovely home.

The young lady had been deep in thought as she dug at the offending weeds that poked out from the gravel. She had a special tool for the task, together with a tin bucket and she squatted as she worked. The weeds came out easily and she knew that the task would be completed in an hour or so.

Someone wolf-whistled. It was cheeky and it was piercing. She quickly looked around to see who was being flattered and who was doing the whistling. There stood her prince from the dance hall. The man of her dreams. Handsome and happy and with a neatly trimmed moustache. Dressed this time, not in a suit, but in paint spattered dove-grey overalls and wearing a huge smile and sparkling hazel eyes. He threw back his head, his hands on his waist, and laughed at her expression and pretty blush. Shirley was speechless and clumsy in her embarrassment, knocking over the bucket of weeds and then falling back off her haunches and on to her bottom, on the gravel.

'Prince Charming' rushed to 'Cinderella's' aid, introducing himself as Burt and offering his hand to help her up from her uncomfortable seat on the gravel.

"What is your name, pretty one?" he asked.

"Sh -Sh- Shirley," she stammered.

"Sh -Sh -Shirley is it?" he teased. "Well, that's the first time I've heard that one."

Shirley pushed his arm lightly, correcting him with a smile on her face.

"No s-silly. It's just Shirley."

"Tell me 'Just Shirley,' are you the mistress of this grand house?"

"No, of course not. I'm just the maid.....who sometimes does odd jobs like the weeding. But I do live here."

She looked up at him through her curls, giving him her prettiest smile.

"And do you ever go dancing as well, Shirley the pretty maid."

He winked at her and gave her his one eye brow raised most handsome Clark Gable impersonation.

She almost fainted!

"Yes I do. I have seen you at The Embassy.

Shirley suddenly blushed, putting her hands over her mouth as if she had said something wrong.

"Aha. You have noticed me. I am flattered. Do you want to go with me one night, Shirley?"

The sixteen year old was unfamiliar with young men and dating and felt overwhelmed, but pleased. *He must be one of the painters. Fancy him turning up at her place of employment. He had asked her out, and he had only seen her in her maid's outfit. Wait until he saw her in her lovely new dress.* Her heart was pounding with excitement.

Someone called out to Burt to come and earn his pay and he started to move off.

"Are you one of the painters?" she forced herself to ask him a question.

"I was helping out my brother Jack and our father with a couple of painting jobs, but I have just finished up at trade school. I am now a master plumber. They needed a plumber here, so I will fix the problem and then give Jack and Dad a hand with the painting."

Burt could not keep the pride out of his voice. He had worked very hard and had to pay his own way, studying and working at the same time. He also supported both of his parents by paying their rent, so he was not afraid of hard work and was a good and generous manager.

Realising that he would be gone in a few seconds, her courage rose and she answered his question.

"Yes." She blurted out the word. "Yes. I mean...." Nothing came to her. "Yes," she said again and then looked down shyly.

He winked at her again, as he moved away.

"I'll call for you Shirley. Next Saturday night. Expect me around seven."

He ran down the driveway and disappeared around the back of the house.

She stood there staring down the driveway, hoping for another glimpse of him.

Am I dreaming? Did that just happen? Did he just ask me to go the dance with him? That's too amazing. I see him at the dance. I get a crush on him and then he turns up at the very house where I am living and working. Did the Lord do that? Was that you Jesus? Did you answer my prayer and send

Someone to Watch Over Me

someone to care for me? Is this the beginning of something special? Thank you. Thank you so much. This must be you at work. I have goose bumps all over. I feel it is you. And I now have a beautiful dress to wear - in the nick of time. It has all come together. It must be you at work, answering my prayers.

Shirley was literally skipping now towards the side door.

I must find Mrs. Brogan and tell her what just happened. She will be amazed too. Maybe she can convince Mr. Brogan to give me a few dance lessons. Burt is so good. I can't have him thinking I am a dumb-cluck on the dance floor.

The ecstatic girl skipped through the house, towards the kitchen, bursting to tell her good news.

Someone to Watch Over Me

Chapter Forty Two

"Adversity is like a strong wind. It tears away from us all but the things that cannot be torn, so that we see ourselves as we really are."   Arthur Goden, 'Memoirs of a Geisha'

Burt met Shirley when their country was at war. It was a very dark time, but life went on as Australians tried to forget the horrors of war, reminding themselves that it was a long way away and would hopefully end soon.

They ate meagrely, food now being rationed, worked when it was available, played cards, danced, went to the picture theatre, made love, laughed and cried, much the same as before the war. The gloomy shadow of war hung like a black cloud over everything, but the resilience of the Aussie spirit rose above the gloom, despite bad news.

World War Two ran from September 1st, 1939 until September 2nd, 1945 where, tragically, over sixty million people were killed. Some estimate the numbers as closer to eighty million. Whatever the number of lives lost, they represented individuals who were loved and missed. They represented families who grieved the loss of their loved ones and who struggled to accept the huge waste of young lives. Much hardship was the dreadful legacy of the war years, resulting in poverty and shortage of food supplies. Rationing of tea, butter, sugar, clothing and shoes became necessary. The Nation was gripped with fear as to when and how the war would end.

Someone to Watch Over Me

Women were encouraged to work in factories and fill the gaps left by the men who had gone to fight for their country. Many women responded to this urgent need and the numbers of females joining the workforce were greatly increased.

Compulsory military service, called conscription, came into force in 1943. By September, 1945, when the war ended, one million men and women had decided to fight for their country. One thousand people were sadly prosecuted for taking their stand as conscientious objectors. Some found themselves imprisoned for this action.

Life continued being played out against this trying backdrop. It was hard for everyone.

It was even harder for some. Burt's father, Walter was a chronic alcoholic, and the faster Burt made money the quicker it disappeared. He resorted to bringing home supplies, when he could get hold of them, instead of cash. It seemed that wherever he hid the money, his father could sniff it out. Money was just too hard to come by to lose it to his father's addiction, so Burt eventually carried whatever money he had, on his person.

He was extremely creative, an amateur artist, and always trying to come up with new ideas to survive their poverty. He would paint exquisite wooden brooches. He painted pictures of people's houses on these oval-shaped wooden pieces and then endeavoured to sell them door to door, to the more wealthy home owners. He sold a few, but it was not easy. Money was tight.

He rode his bike up into the Adelaide Hills and dug for gold. He had a romantic idea of digging up a nugget and becoming rich. He actually managed to find a few specks of gold and these were kept in a small glass bottle with a wax seal, to remind him of one phase of his life. Walter, Jack and Burt painted and decorated houses as the Clough Team, when the work came in. They liked to call themselves "the Cloughies," Jack being Burt's older brother. They would walk around the district, knocking on doors, trying to find work. Burt offered his services, also, as a master plumber, and took on whatever work was available no matter how difficult. He could not believe one job, when he had to find a man's false teeth which had disappeared down the toilet. He eventually located them, his stomach turning over as he handed them to their owner. He did not want to know if the man was going to wear them again.

Burt was embarrassed that he had not gone to war to fight for his country. He was no coward, and would have willingly gone, had he been accepted. He would have taken on any enemy and fought well. He was a fighter by nature - fighting all sorts of hardships daily, and standing nose to nose with any aggressor. However, he was not accepted into the army because he was a qualified tradesman. Tradesmen were needed to keep things in order at home.

He had been seriously ill with bacterial meningitis two years before and had almost died. His doctor told him the condition is sometimes fatal and can cause serious long-term complications. Burt was lucky. He had been hospitalised for quite a long time but the medical staff had brought him through. He had, however, been left with impaired hearing. This and the uncertain prognosis in regard to long term effects of the illness caused him to think that he may be rejected as a possible recruit for the services. However, to be rejected because he was a tradesman really upset him. He thought that no-one would believe that he was unacceptable because of his trade. He was devastated and applied again, only to be told he was needed at home because he was a qualified tradesman. Sometimes Burt romanced about how he could hide his identity and get accepted, but nothing ever eventuated. Meanwhile he felt guilty that others were fighting overseas and here he was, a relatively fit and healthy male, looking like a coward. Many other men were rejected too and also had to cope with the accusations, imagined or real.

Someone to Watch Over Me

Burt had learned from a young age, despite his dysfunctional family life, to put on a happy face. He was a charming, fun-loving young man and always the life of a party. He was popular with everyone, except when someone got on the wrong side of him, and then he knew how to defend himself or someone else. He would threaten to 'knock their block off' if they crossed him, or offended someone he cared about. He needed the right woman to tame him. He was looking for someone to love, to protect and to shower with affection. He was passionate and he was lonely. He wanted someone who was teachable. He had some low self-esteem issues and wanted a partner who needed to be rescued and who would see him as their hero. He had been engaged to a local girl from down the street, but had broken the engagement with Kathleen when she disappointed him with a temper tantrum. Perhaps she reminded him too much of his mother, Margaret, who was unequalled with her merciless outbursts and uncontrolled tongue. He wanted someone who looked up to him and appreciated him and whom he could protect and comfort. The die was cast. His home life had consisted of raging, violent fights and hurtful, unkind words. He had seen his father brow-beaten by a much taller and domineering woman every day of his life.

Burt was looking for someone needy and unprotected, just like Shirley Gilfillan. Someone to play heroine to his hero. A damsel in distress for Clark Gable to rescue and adore.

Chapter Forty Three

"Joy is the feeling of grinning on the inside." Dr. Melba Colgrove

Her thoughtful employer had given her an 'early minute' so that she could spend extra time preening and fussing for her dance date, and especially for Burt. Extra dance tuition had been given by the kindly Mr. Brogan, who had taken an instant liking to Burton James. He hoped that the young folk would have a good time together. His old heart had been warmed to see their maid's unbridled joy. He had been impressed with how quickly Shirley had picked up the steps to all the dances he knew. He and Mrs. Brogan were sitting at the kitchen table, enjoying a cup of tea and awaiting the transformed appearance of their maid. She was still behind the door, in her tiny bedroom.

There was a knock on the front door. Mr. Brogan went to open it and Mrs. Brogan quickly tapped on Shirley's door to alert her. Shirley did not answer. Her employer knocked again, calling out her name this time. Not receiving an answer, the older woman slowly opened the door, fearful that shy Shirley may have been overcome with nerves, and bolted out the window, or worse still, fainted.

The girl was standing, frozen to the spot, eyeing herself in the small mirror, and examining herself with a definite frown.

"Whatever is the matter? You look absolutely lovely, and your young man is waiting in the hallway. What is keeping you for goodness sake?"

Shirley shook her head in disagreement.

"I don't look very nice at all. He will notice my blind eye. I am not very good at dancing and my dress is too fussy and my hair is mousy brown. He is gorgeous and I am plain.....aren't I?"

A tear rolled slowly down her cheek, and then another.

Mrs. Brogan knew just what Shirley needed right now. A good, firm, motherly piece of advice.

"You do not have time for this rubbish young lady. You look lovely, you dance reasonably well, and will continue to improve with practice, your dress is very pretty, it suits you well and your hair is shiny and curly and attractive. You are not plain, but lovely. Burt obviously thinks so, because he has noticed you and asked you to a dance. What are you standing here for like a foolish, empty-headed child? Get out there and let him be the judge as to how you look. I think that will make you feel better. You just have a bit of stage-fright, that's all."

The sixteen year old seemed to see the sense of the straight talk from Mrs. Brogan. She grabbed her clutch bag and wrap from her bed, opened her door and walked quickly into the hallway, giving her employer a hint of a smile as she went.

When Burt saw her, his eyes shone and he wolf-whistled, again. Nothing more needed to be said other than polite 'good nights' as they walked off through the front door together, chatting and laughing at something the young man said. He had borrowed his friend's utility and he carefully arranged a rug on the front seat to keep her dress clean. Having assisted her into the cabin, he then walked around the utility, whistling to himself a popular tune as he slid into the seat next to his date. Shirley was to discover that Burt often whistled to cover his own nervousness. He had learned this habit from one of his film-star heroes in a movie and it seemed to be a good cover for low-self esteem.

They had a wonderful time. She was the envy of every girl in the dance hall. Especially Ida, who kept glaring at her whenever she looked anxiously in her direction. Apparently, Burt had taken

Someone to Watch Over Me

Ida out a few times, and asked her to be his regular dance partner. When he and Shirley arrived at The Embassy, he had excused himself for a moment and taken Ida aside, explaining to her that things had changed. He pointed out that he had a new dance partner and he apologised. Ida was furious as she had been hopeful of something permanent with Burt.

Shirley could not help feeling pleased with herself, even though she felt sorry for Ida. She knew that Ida was an amazing dancer and marvelled at her luck that Burt would drop her for his date with Shirley. They had every dance together, and throughout the night he whispered little tips to help her. She listened to everything he said, and by the end of the night she had improved admirably. He had a disarming way of making her laugh at herself whenever she forgot and looked at her feet, or counted to the music. When she relaxed in his arms and let him lead her, they floated around the floor as if they had been dancing together for years.

All too soon the last dance was announced and they danced, oblivious to everyone else on the floor. When it came to an end, Burt fetched her wrap and clutch bag from her chair and escorted her to his borrowed car. Her head was in the clouds as she took his arm and noticed the other girls looking at her in awe. He was twenty nine years old. This she had discovered about him while they danced. He was almost twice her age, but he was full of energy and fun and seemed much younger. She felt so grown up with him. He was a man of the world, and knew so much. She felt secure with him. He treated her with respect and made her heart race.

When they arrived back at the Brogan's place, he slowed the car down and parked at the entrance to their driveway. Shirley had loved the way he had flirted with her at the dance, twirling her hair around his fingers and letting the curls spring back into place. He had almost kissed her on the dance floor. She was aglow with youthful passion and hoped he would kiss her goodnight, like she saw in the movies.

They sat in the cabin of the utility and he reached his arm around her shoulder, drawing her closer to him. Shirley was certain that he would hear her heart pounding. Very slowly he leaned towards her, gently brushing her lips with his. Then again, and again. Then he kissed her hard and passionately, holding her close to his heart. She was shy, but she was passionate, too, and she kissed him back, hard and long. She had learned a lot from him already. He cupped her chin in his hands, looking deep into her blue eyes and whispering endearments that she had never heard before. He called her 'darling' and 'pretty one' and praised her for how well she had danced and what great company she had been. He asked her to go to the dance with him again the following week and she had sighed her reply as she nodded her head to punctuate her "yes."

Finally, she thought that she had better go, so she pulled herself reluctantly away from his embrace. She was fearful that the Brogans were watching from the window, with the lights turned off, and that she would be reprimanded the next day. She said good-night to him, feeling certain that Burt would have liked her to stay with him longer. She knew that she was smitten and felt that he may be as well. Never before in her life had she received such loving attention. What a dream he was. What an amazing catch for any lucky girl.

But he was HER catch.

HER rescuer.

HER love.

HER Burtie.

Someone to Watch Over Me

Chapter Forty Four

"God, Who began the good work within you, will keep right on helping you grow in His grace until His task within you is finally finished....."   Phillipians 1 : 6 (Living Bible)

As a young man in his early twenties, Burton James Clough loved to brag about being the president of the local Prospect Bachelor's Club. One by one his friends deserted the cause as they married their sweethearts. Burt almost did the same, for a short time, when he became engaged. He had been trying to teach his fiancée Kathleen to drive, but her temper tantrum caused a huge row and he broke the engagement on the spot. He declared himself, once again, the committed president of the diminishing club and a true and grateful bachelor. He determined to evangelise the district, spreading the word of freedom and singlehood.

Burt liked women though. He particularly liked them to be feminine and demure. He had an aversion to women standing with their hands on their hips, or arms folded. He thought that this was unflattering, and demonstrated a haughty and bossy disposition. He had a passion for the movies, just like Shirley did, and he was quite taken with Carole Lombard. He loved her feminine hands and somehow forgave her for her uncouth mouth and down to earth sense of humour. The fact that his look-alike screen idol, Clark Gable, was passionately in love with Carole Lombard, and married her, probably influenced his opinion, profoundly.

Someone to Watch Over Me

Shirley worshipped her Burt. She hung on every word that he uttered. When she discovered his obsession with 'feminine hands,' she practiced in her bedroom mirror until she felt she had mastered control over hers. At no time were her hands allowed to find their way to her hips, or her waist, or her arms to fold in front of her chest. No matter how cold the weather became, her hands remained by her side, or in her pockets. She loved it when she was able to slip one hand into his strong, protective hand. She would warm one hand up in his and then move to his other side and slip her freezing hand into his to warm it up as well.

Burt was out-going, opinionated and popular. His handsome good looks gave him confidence, and he was particular about his clothes. He had a real talent for keeping up with fashion on a meagre income. His wardrobe was limited but sharp. He had started growing a moustache, emulating his idol, and was pleased with the comments that this drew. A cheeky hat at a jaunty angle was his trade mark and he usually had a cigarette hanging from the corner of his mouth. The smoke that drifted up caused his eyes to water a little and close in a sleepy fashion. He decided that this made him look more attractive than ever, so it was worth the discomfort to his poor eyes. Burt preferred to wear fashionable slacks with silky fabric shirts and matching ties. He always looked immaculate, standing out in the crowd and catching the eyes of young women wherever he went. One could be excused for thinking that he came from a well-to-do home, and not the alcoholic, impoverished one in which he actually lived. Perhaps he was influenced by the fact that a distant family member had taken to his older brother Jack and paid all his school fees through Christian Brothers College, a Catholic private school. Jack's friends and associates were of a higher social standing than Burt's and this caused a great chip to form on the younger brother's shoulder. All of his life he disliked people who seemed out of his reach and better off than he, referring to them as snobs.

Someone to Watch Over Me

He managed to fill the gaps in his life with sports, enjoying good success on both the football field and cricket ground. Playing district football he won trophies for fairest and best player and never gave anything but his best during the matches. The lack of family funds handicapped his cricket opportunities, but he won several trophies, playing district cricket for Prospect. It was during that era in which the great Don Bradman began his career and for the rest of his life he told the story of how he clean-bowled Sir Don during one match. He was very proud of the different cups and trophies he won at his beloved sports.

Burt loved his parents dearly. He somehow managed to overlook their obvious faults and limitations and treated them with great respect. His siblings saw him as the one with the responsibility to look after their parents, and abandoned him to the task. The only way he could afford to do this was for them to live with him, saving them the need to rent another house. He despaired at his father's heavy drinking, but had tried, and failed, to get him to stop.

Burt had a conversion experience as a teenager. His family was Catholic, but, somehow, Burt found himself in a Protestant church, looking for some answers to his many questions. It was Prospect Church of Christ. He was searching for some light to shine into his very grey existence with his parents, with poverty, and a broken heart and a tragic world war. One of his mates was a Christian and he had invited him along to his church. Burt listened with open ears to words that broke into his discouragement like sunrise across the darkened earth. He heard that God loved Him, Jesus had died to take the punishment for his wrong-doing and that the Holy Spirit could empower him.

He rose from his pew and walked to the front of the church while the choir sang *'Just as I Am.'* The minister shook his hand and welcomed him into the family of God. Burt's face was wet with tears as he came alive to a new faith and family.

Someone to Watch Over Me

Young Burt was always enthusiastic and conscientious and now he had a new direction for his life. He threw himself into the service of the church, enthusiastically adjusting to the new culture and vocabulary. He was quickly established in the Sunday school as a new teacher and the young boys in his class hung on his sporting adventure stories. He developed a deep love for the Bible and read it, learning his favourite verses off by heart.

His passion for teaching rose to the surface and he started to think about going into the ministry as a Church of Christ minister, much to the chagrin of Margaret and Walter, who would have rather seen him a priest in the Catholic faith. Many arguments ensued, but Burt did his best to respect his parents, requesting that they in turn respect his rights to his own decisions. He had been running a Saturday night dance at the local Masonic hall for a year or two. The Churches of Christ at Prospect frowned on dancing and this caused Burt to fall out of favour with some of the leaders in his church. He was instructed to close the dance down, as some of the church young people attended and were sometimes late for church, or did not turn up at all. Burt was shocked and angry. He stood his ground and was shut out from the church community not long after he was welcomed into the church.

This rejection hurt him deeply and he kept away from churches for twenty four years. Strangely enough, it was another Church of Christ, at Nailsworth, which brought healing to the deep wound in his spirit. Once again he walked to the front of the church while the choir sang, this time a children's Sunday school anniversary choir. Two of his daughters came down from the steep platform, which held approximately two hundred children, They were taking an expected stand to demonstrate their new found faith in God. Father and daughters stood together, his girls not fully understanding the huge impact that this experience had on their father.

Someone to Watch Over Me

He was quickly welcomed and accepted into the church family and elected to the church board. His passion for Bible reading never waned. He had a great Bible knowledge throughout his lifetime, and this caused some interesting debates with ministers whom Burt thought were giving incorrect interpretations of Scripture.

Whatever Burt took on, he threw himself into it with enthusiasm and fervour. He brought these qualities to his friendship with the young Shirley. He was thirteen years older than her, but this meant that he could teach her about the world, and protect her from it.

He could try, anyway.

Chapter Forty Five

"Your worst days are never so bad that you are beyond the reach of God's grace. And your best days are never so good that you are beyond the need of God's grace." Terry Bridges

Shirley and Burt had been seeing each other for a few weeks when Burt told her that he was taking her to Sunday lunch at his parent's place. Shirley was both excited and nervous. The street-wise girl had wondered why her boy-friend had taken so long to invite her home to meet his parents. She guessed that they were not too happy with his relationship with her. Or, on the other hand, she guessed that he was not too proud of them and worried about how they might behave towards her. They lived very near to the Brogan's, so the couple walked together, Burt having walked to collect her.

He had picked some flowers along the way, and he held them out to her with a kiss on her cheek. She had waited for him in the front garden and shyly received his carefree little bunch of violets, noticing the beautiful perfume as she held the flowers to her nose.

As they walked along, he chatted with her about his parents, Margaret and Walter Clough, his brother Jack and his sisters Ella and Rose. Burt was the baby of the family and the responsibility for his parents seemed to rest on his shoulders. In no time at all they arrived at the house in Boyle Street, Prospect and Shirley was impressed, straight away, with the lovely rose arch in the tiny

Someone to Watch Over Me

front garden. It was covered with deep burgundy and velvety roses that made an amazing display, filling the short walk to the front door. It was a little overgrown, but it made a warm welcome to anyone visiting the Clough home. Shirley took this as a good sign of things to come. She guessed that someone in the house must be a keen gardener and knew instantly that it was her Burtie.

He walked her proudly to the front door, whistling as they went. She recognised the tune as a hit number that the popular Andrews Sisters sang, *'Don't sit Under the Apple Tree'*[5] and quietly sang a few bars for him. It was the first time he had heard her sing. He was speechless and stopped walking, turning to look at her with a shocked look on his face. He recognised that she had a beautiful voice and also perfect pitch. He started whistling a couple more lines to coach her to sing again, but the impromptu moment had gone and she refused to co-operate. He made a mental note to try to get her to sing later on. He knew a sensational voice when he heard one.

As he opened the front door, he called out that they had arrived. Ushering Shirley past the front room, he steered her to where he knew his parents would be, in the kitchen. He grimaced as he noticed how untidy the house was and how it must look through Shirley's eyes. There was stuff everywhere. Every seat or table or cupboard had something piled high on it. There were boxes everywhere and old newspapers and magazines stacked up on the floor and against the walls. Clean washing, not yet folded or put away, spread itself out across the settee in the front room, so there would have been nowhere at all for them to sit. He kept walking, pulling Shirley along with him, hoping that the kitchen would be more presentable.

Shirley was shocked at the over cluttered home, but mostly because memories had just been triggered of her own mother's

---

[5] From the movie "Private Buckeroo." Composed by Sam H. Stept and lyrics by Lew Brown and Charles Tobias

untidy and disordered house. She had suddenly been transported back to the night when the two police officers had come to her door and eventually taken her from her mother. She remembered the feeling of shame as they looked around with disdain at the mess and grubbiness everywhere in the house that had been her home.

Instinctively Shirley realised that Burt felt shame at the state of his home. She could tell that he was deeply disappointed and guessed that he had asked them to tidy up for today, especially. She moved closer to him and gave him an encouraging squeeze on his hand.

"I love the rose arch out front. Did you do that?"

She wanted to make him feel better.

"Yes. I could tell that you liked it."

He squeezed her hand back, cheering up a little.

They arrived at the kitchen and there sat Burt's father, already 'under the weather' in his usual chair at the head of the incredibly cluttered table. He didn't even look at Shirley or greet his benevolent son. He sat staring into space, his glass of beer clutched in his right hand and his left draped around a large bottle of beer. Shirley noticed that the bottle was almost empty and wondered how long ago he'd started on it. She glanced over at the wood stove where Burt's mother stood, stirring something in an over-sized, blackened pot, with a very large wooden paddle, scowling in their direction.

Burt cheerfully did the introductions and asked a friendly question.

"What's for lunch, Mum? Smells wonderful. You always were a marvellous cook. So is Shirley, you know. She's cooking at the place where she boards."

The younger woman tried to smile at the older one. She noticed that she was dressed entirely in black. Her long skirt almost reached her thick black socks which gathered around her ankles. She noticed the tops of the socks had been cut with scissors and that the older woman's legs were very swollen, looking straight up and down without any shape where her ankles should be. On her very large feet were men's slippers, which had also been cut to accommodate her swollen feet. She wore a huge black shirt over her skirt and her steel grey hair was extremely long and pulled back with a rubber band at the nape of her neck. As she stood stirring the concoction on the stove, Shirley stood staring at what she thought was a perfect caricature of a witch.

My Burt's mother is a witch, she thought to herself, shocked. *Burt's father is a drunk,* followed, in her thoughts.

Without thinking, she nestled closer to Burt and felt his protective arm go around her shoulders, seeming to tune into her thoughts.

The older woman looked her up and down in the awkward silence. Her eyes settled on the small bunch of violets that she clutched tightly.

"Who are they for?" came the words in her direction, like a slap across her face.

"B-B-Burt picked them for m-m-me," was all that she could think to say.

"Give them to me you stupid girl. The way you're squeezing them, they'll be dead in no time." Margaret reached out and grabbed the flowers from the frightened girl and then filled a jar full of water from the tap and placed the violets in the jar, squeezing the jar amongst the clutter on the window sill. Somehow Shirley knew that this stranger would not return her flowers when it was time for her to leave this strange house. She was right.

She offered to set the table, to help with lunch, but when she looked at the table, there was no room for anything else. Walter had the Sunday paper the Sunday Mail spread out over everything, and things like various jams and honey and treacle, Bonox, Vegemite, tomato sauce, salt and pepper, sugar and a huge jar of home-pickled onions seemed to be always left out on the old rickety wooden table, together with newspaper cuttings, stacks of used envelopes and other bits and pieces. Across the room several lengths of string were strung, and pegs clipped newspaper cuttings, aged by the years, to the strings.

Shirley saw the comic page and glanced at Ginger Meggs. She remembered those treasured Sundays with Charlie reading the comic strip to her with different voices to suit the different characters. This was her main introduction to reading. It had left an impression to last a life-time. As she sadly remembered her beloved uncle, recalling how he called her his little 'side-kick', she wondered where on earth he was now. It had been years since she had any contact with him. She remembered one time when he had called on her at the orphanage, taking her for a walk down on the beach at Largs Bay. He'd brought an aboriginal spear to show her, from 'up north' where he'd been working. He also had a banana in his cardigan pocket, which he had given her to eat. She had hungrily devoured it, including the skin. It was the first piece of fruit that she had eaten in a very long time. She asked herself, now, if he had noticed that she was starving, and if he cared.

The crabby old woman brought her back from her daydreaming by dismissing her offer of help and ordering the young couple outside until she called them for lunch. Shirley and Burt gratefully escaped the tension for awhile and amused themselves checking out all of the different plants that were haphazardly planted in pots, old baths, tea-pots, chipped china bowls, enamel basins and all sorts of interesting containers. Shirley especially liked looking at the chipped jugs and tea-pots which held various miniature cacti. It was the most interesting garden she had ever seen and the huge variety of plants added to the appeal. A few fruit trees towered over geraniums, which splashed reds, pinks and mauves all over the garden. Pelargoniums seemed to thrive as well, competing with the geraniums for attention.

"How gorgeous!" shrieked Shirley, spell-bound.

Someone to Watch Over Me

She skirted the flower beds with their tidy edging of pieces of timber, or old house bricks with their corners sitting up proudly, creating a lovely patterned edging. She gasped at the neat vegetable garden, proudly showing off its rhubarb, potatoes, spinach, sweet corn, staked tomatoes, beans on a trellis and pumpkins wandering freely all over the place.

Burt observed her excited reaction with pride. He had worked very hard to keep their garden under control and to grow vegetables to keep them fed as cheaply as possible. He was rightfully proud of his efforts and it all seemed worthwhile to be rewarded by her pleasure.

"I'm glad you appreciate my little hobby. I think we're having vegetable soup for lunch, straight out of my garden. What do you think of that now, young lady?"

"I think it's something to be very proud of young man," she said with a giggle, running off and encouraging him to chase her around the flower beds.

As he laughed and chased her, Burt now found his mind going to the end of each day, when he came home from work and went straight out into his garden, before sunset. His father would spend the whole day at the 'pub' and his mother would go to fetch him and bring him home for the evening meal. It was a pitiful sight, but no-one seemed to know what to do about it. Walter became violent when approached about his drinking and would hit Margaret, beating her until she was badly bruised. He was much shorter than his wife, but a force to be reckoned with when drunk. When he was sober, no-one wanted to disturb the cherished peace and so his ugly addiction went unmentioned. The anger and resentment, however, came out in other directions and Margaret was always extremely grumpy, nagging him and paying him back by making his life as miserable as he made hers.

The back door flew open, bringing Burt back to the present moment.

Someone to Watch Over Me

"Come on. Are you deaf or something? Lunch is ready. Come now or eat it cold. It's up to you."

Margaret went back into the house, banging the screen door behind her.

Someone to Watch Over Me

Chapter Forty Six

"Who will tell whether one happy moment of love, or the joy of breathing, or walking on a bright morning and smelling the fresh air, is not worth all the suffering and effort which life implies." Eric Fromm

She was in love and she wanted his mother to love her too. She did everything but turn herself inside out to win the approval of the other woman. She was beginning to see that her mission was futile. Her enemy was the jealousy of a woman who was not prepared to share her son's affection.

Diligently her surplus pennies were stored away like a squirrel's cache of nuts for the winter. Her plan was conceived from something she saw in a Greer Garson movie. If she gave her enemy a beautiful gift, then they may be able to bury the hatchet and become friends. It did not occur to her in her inexperience that she may be judged as trying to 'buy' acceptance. It took her quite a few weeks, but eventually she had enough money saved up to purchase her surprise gift for Margaret Clough. She hurried up Rundle Street in the city on a mission that gave her hope and pleasure.

After much deliberation, she settled on a pretty, sparkly brooch from Woolworths. She carefully wrapped her gift in some tissue paper and tied it up with blue hair ribbon, left over from the Alice head band she had made. Shirley presented it nervously to Burt's mother, holding her breath with anticipation, hopeful of some warmth and appreciation.

Someone to Watch Over Me

"What's this all about? Hrmph. Been out wasting money have we young lady. I don't need your gifts...common sense is what I'd like to see from you. You'll have to grow up before that happens, I suspect."

She snorted as she undid the ribbon and tissue paper and after glaring at the pretty brooch, handed it back to the disappointed girl with a grunt of disapproval.

The rejection of her gift mirrored the rejection of herself by this cruel woman who may have been a much needed mother in Shirley's deprived life. The young woman stood there with tears running down her face, struggling to work out what she had done wrong, while determining to find a way to win this woman's affection and acceptance. Her hunger prevailed and she worked hard whenever she visited Burt's home.

Somehow her script for life dictated that hard sacrificial work would make her a worthwhile person. Sadly, his parents were not capable of giving to her what she needed and deserved. Burt was nothing like either of his mean-spirited parents and over-compensated with everyone, trying to make up for their lack.

Finally, Shirley gave up trying to please them and decided just to concentrate on pleasing their son. Margaret became angry and resentful towards them, detesting having to spend time with them in order to spend time with him. The young couple would catch up with each other whenever they could and avoided Margaret and Walter whenever possible as well.

Their circle of friends and contacts grew as did their love for each other. Shirley smiled to herself when she saw in Burton James the 'someone to watch over her' that she had always yearned for.

Chapter Forty Seven

"O Lord, you have examined my heart and know everything about me. You know when I sit or stand. When far away, you know my every thought. You chart the path ahead of me, and tell me where to stop and rest. Every moment you know where I am. You know what I am going to say before I even say it. You both precede and follow me, and place your hand of blessing on my head."

Psalm 139 verses 1 - 5.
Living Bible.

Shirley felt ill. Eating her breakfast was out of the question. She rushed to the toilet and vomited, at just the thought of food. She was irritable and would cry over nothing. This went on for days and she was worried. Her 'girl friend', as she called her monthly period, didn't turn up. She had to see Burt. He loved her too, she knew that. Just last week he had told her, and she'd cried. He told her that he had a pain in his chest when he thought about her and he knew it wasn't indigestion but love. They had both laughed.

"I know that people have treated you badly, Shirl. Your heart is bruised and battered. I want to look after you and keep you safe. I want to kiss away all that pain. I want to make up to you for all the abuse and rejection that has been so unfairly hurled at you. I love you so much."

Someone to Watch Over Me

His words mixed with her tears as they held each other, determining to weather together whatever storms would be on their path ahead.

Shirley knew she had to talk with him about her suspicions of an ensuing storm of mammoth proportions. She hoped he had meant his words and that he would want to rescue her from this next difficult challenge.

"I'm a good girl. A good girl. The nuns said God would punish me for this sin that Burt and I have committed. This would make me a bad girl. I would not be fit for heaven. I would be rejected by Jesus. He would not want a bad girl. I must do something. Where will I live? What will I do? I can't board and work as a maid. No-one will want a single pregnant girl living in and working for them. What have I done. If no-one knows and I get rid of this poor baby then life can go on. Burt may not want me when he knows. This is a disaster. I must do something. I am in big trouble."

Shirley cried into her pillow and worried all night, tossing and turning on her bed. She had a plan. First she must see a doctor and confirm if she was pregnant. Then she would decide what to do.

As soon as she had some time off, Shirley rode her bike to the doctor's surgery and made an urgent appointment.

"Shirley, I know you are very worried and I wish I could give you the answer that you want. I am afraid, though that you are expecting a baby."

The kindly doctor looked at her over the top of his glasses while putting a reassuring hand on her shoulder. He clearly understood that this was a huge dilemma for the sixteen year old. The distressed girl left his surgery in tears.

Shirley contacted a couple of her old friends who had talked about a self-aborting method and asked them for details. It involved using a knitting needle. They warned her that some women had died trying this method. She was desperate. She prepared herself and started the procedure. Bursting into tears the distressed young girl threw the knitting needle across the room and herself on her bed. She would not do this. This baby deserved to live. She would not put her own needs before this little baby whom she and Burt had made together. She must talk with Burt. He was a good man. He loved her. He would have a solution.

Finally they caught up on the phone. She told him that she needed to see him urgently. He explained that he would be across town working on a house, as a plumber this time, and wouldn't be able to see her for a couple of days. He said if he could possibly get away he would, but he didn't like his chances.

Shirley watched for him for two days. Between chores she would go out to the front of the house and watch up the road for him. She loved the way he nonchalantly sauntered along, hat tipped back on his head, hands in his pockets and always whistling a tune. She longed for this now. Her Burtie. He would understand. He would rescue her. He would know what to do.

When she heard the hall clock chime 5 o'clock on the second day, she broke down again, her face in her hands as she sat on her bed in her yellow room. Her sobs shook her body as fresh realisation of her desperate situation engulfed her. Who could she run to? What could a lonely, penniless girl do in her situation? Her present accommodation was for a working girl, not a pregnant child of sixteen. If the Brogans found out, they would turn her out, as nice as they were. Her own father had heartlessly abandoned her when she was a tiny child. How could she trust him to give her any support now that she had a child on the way? Money was a huge issue to him as he did not have a home of his own, but lived with Molly and her mother in their rented home. They had taken him in as a boarder to help their financial plight. It was hard times. The two women had shared the double bed to clear a room for him, so it was hard to see how Shirley and her baby could fit into the small place as well.

Someone to Watch Over Me

Charlie. There was always Charlie. She had found him recently. She had forgiven him for abandoning her and they were friends again. Would he help her now that she had made such a mess of things? He had never married. She had never known him to even have a woman friend, or to go on a date of any kind. He had told her that he'd been put off women years ago. She remembered a terrible scene when Phyllis had been allowed to leave the mental institution at Parkside for a weekend home visit, with Charlie and Shirley. Phyllis had drunk a lot from his flagon of sherry and had disgraced herself with her out of control behaviour. Shirley vaguely remembered the noisy and heated argument between brother and sister. The raised voices and accusations flew back and forth and the frightened child ran and hid under her bed. Her mother was screeching and throwing things and banging doors and breaking everything in sight. Phyllis said some awful things to Charlie and hurt him deeply. This had been a turning point for him, revealing that his sister was never going to be capable of looking after her only child. He felt tricked and trapped. He could tell she was getting worse and not better as he had hoped.

Without the alcohol she was crazy enough, but she seemed to have no control of her drinking if there was any alcohol in sight. Shirley remembered the silence from then on in regard to his sister. He never mentioned her, or visited her as he used to at Parkside Mental Hospital. Sadly, he too drank too much these days. He was lonely and sad and disappointed. Life's sorrow had brought him to his knees. He was 'broke'. He was also broken.

The pregnant young girl could not see him helping her and her baby as he had helped her all those years ago. She became frantic. There seemed to be nowhere to turn. Where was Burt? What had happened to him? He knew she needed to speak with him urgently. Had he decided to listen to his nasty mother after all and dump her? Had he fallen for someone else? Someone smart and pretty and with two good eyes? She fell back on her

Someone to Watch Over Me

bed in despair. Staring at the ceiling, searching for an answer, tears trickled from the corners of her worried eyes and made their way down the edges of her face, on to her pillow.

Chapter Forty Eight

"You were there while I was being formed in utter seclusion! You saw me before I was born and scheduled each day of my life before I began to breathe."
Psalm 139 verses 15 and 16.
The Living Bible

A whole week had gone by with no word from the father of her hidden, terrible secret. She had decided to tell no-one until she had a chance to talk with Burt. Several times she'd come close to trying laxatives to abort her baby, and then borrowed a knitting needle from Mrs. Brogan's knitting basket in the sitting room. Very quickly, however, she had returned it to its usual place and hurried back to her duties. She had heard the stories of the girls who'd panicked and tried to get rid of their babies in this way, and that they'd either damaged themselves permanently, or even died. She knew God would not approve either and once again resigned herself to her plight. Being pregnant was a desperate plight indeed in those days, without much support or compassion, but with much pointing of fingers.

The week-end finally arrived and on Saturday afternoon, so did Burt. He explained that he had been away unexpectedly on a painting job straight after the plumbing one, as his brother and father needed his help and also the money. It was a big undertaking and required the three men to complete it within a tight deadline. It was an old farmhouse in Mannum, east of

Someone to Watch Over Me

Adelaide on the River Murray and it badly needed freshening up for a wedding.

"You'd have loved it Shirley. We had to cross over the river on a punt and then find this place from a map that the people..., hey, whatever is the matter Shirley? You look like something terrible has happened. Has someone treated you badly? Just tell me who and I'll knock their block off! Tell me what's been going on."

He quickly took her hand and led her out the front gate and down the road. When they were a safe distance from the house, Shirley blurted out her problem.

"I'm pregnant, Burt."

She could not look into his eyes, because she was certain he would despise her. Shame enveloped her. She had been stupid. Why didn't she do what the nuns had driven into her and been a 'good girl?'

Why hadn't Burt said something? He was going to walk away and leave her, she knew it. He would not want to be tied down with a young girl and her unwanted baby. He loved his football and his cricket and his bachelor club, and he was already supporting his parents.

Burt took the cigarette from the corner of his mouth and dropped it in the dirt. He stamped it out with his polished shoe as he thoughtfully stroked his chin. He had been shocked at her life-shattering news, but was now processing the facts. He was a problem solver by nature and had a disarming knack of looking on the bright side of things. He was adding things up and working on a solution for their dilemma.

I'll do the right thing by this girl and our baby. After all, I'm twenty nine years old and it's about time I settled down. I love her for Pete's sake. I'll do the honourable thing and marry her. If we tie the knot fast enough, no-one need know she was pregnant at the time. We could use the excuse that Shirley had no family to speak of and needed to move in with me and my parents. That they'd only agree to this if we were married.

Shirley stood there, like a statue, waiting for his response and dreading the worse possible outcome.

"You're going to drop me, aren't you? Everyone will know why! I'm going to get rid of it!"

She burst into tears.

"No-one is going to ask you to. It's my baby too, Shirley."

He put his arms around her trembling body and drew her into his life forever.

"Listen to me, girl. Everything is going to be all right. I will arrange for us to get married straight away and no-one will even know that you are pregnant until we've been married for a few months. We can say we have a honeymoon baby on the way."

They stood there in a tight embrace and then he spoke again, pulling her away from him so he could look into her eyes.

"Have you told anyone yet?"

She shook her head. "Only the doctor knows."

"Good girl. Let's keep it that way. This is no-one else's business but ours. I'll make the arrangements. You work out just who you want at the wedding. Only a couple of people. I'll work out the church. I know you'll want it to be Catholic. I'll arrange somewhere special for our wedding night. There's no way I'm taking you back to my place with my parents there. Plenty of time for that later, as we'll need for you to move into my room with me until I can save up a bit. Then we'll get our own place. Sorry love, but we will make it work. I'll have a talk with Mum and Dad."

All the time he was speaking, Shirley could not believe her ears. In her mind, she was thinking, *He is going to stay with me. He is going to marry me and look after me and the baby. I will have somewhere to live. Eventually we will have our own place. He is working it all out and caring about me.*

The relief overwhelmed her and she felt light in the head and almost fainted. He quickly caught her as her legs gave out and she collapsed. He carried her into the shade of a peppercorn tree in the side street, cradling her in his muscular arms until she was fully conscious again.

"We'd better look after you and our little bubs. We're a family now and you will soon be my wife. I wonder if it's a boy or a girl. Hell's bells. How about that? I'm going to be a father."

He gently put her down on to her feet, steadying her and then holding her against him. They had much to talk about, and many plans to make, and in a huge hurry.

Someone to Watch Over Me

Chapter Forty Nine

"To the world you may be one person, but to one person you may be the world." Bill Wilson

It was a magnificent day. The most beautiful day of her life. Her wedding day. The sun was shining and her heart was dancing. She quickly pulled on her blue suit with the pretty embroidery on three pockets. Her wide brimmed felt hat in a darker blue matched it well and she knew that Burt would like it. Slipping her feet into her black high heels, Shirley picked up her matching black handbag, and Mrs. Noonan's gifted prayer book. Checking her appearance as best she could in the small mirror on her wardrobe door, she decided that she would have to do. There was no money for a wedding dress and veil or a new outfit. This suit had sufficed for meeting up with her father when she was fifteen, and it would do for this other important occasion. Two huge events in her very young life.

She patted her tummy protectively, thinking to herself, *I'm so glad that I didn't get rid of you, but you will need to be a secret for a while yet. Until my tummy pokes out at least. I am not going to tell anyone, no matter how suspicious they are. I saw their looks because everything is so rushed, but if I keep on denying you exist, they will give up in the end. I'll just keep saying that your daddy and I love each other so much that we can't wait to get married and be together. It sounds so romantic. Just like in the movies. His horrid parents won't come to the wedding and have guessed about you, calling me some more nasty names. I wouldn't want them there anyway. My dad and the evil Molly will be there, and Muriel, my friend from St. Jo's. Her sister Anna would have been there, but she's working in the country as a maid and living in with the family. Her sister will do though, even if she is suspicious and asking me lots of questions.*

I am a good girl. I will just pretend that you didn't get started until after I was married. I would never have sex before marriage. The nuns told me how wicked it was and that God would hate me if I did. So I didn't.

Mr and Mrs. Brogan have been very kind to me and wished me well. They looked at me strangely, but I didn't tell them about you. I hate to think that I am going to have to live with Burt's parents for a little while, but he can't turn them out into the street, and he has promised that he will get us a place of our own as soon as he can. That will have to do. It could be worse. Most of my things are at Burt's place already and I will move in there tomorrow.

Shirley was both excited about her wedding and terrified about her living arrangements.

Burt says I am probably under age, so we are going to have to put my age as eighteen on the marriage certificate. He is so clever. He will look after us now. We are going to be a happy family. Shirley hugged herself and smiled at her image in the mirror.

There was a knock on her door.

"Time to go lassie."

Sad farewells were said to her kind employer, Mrs. Brogan, who then surprised her with a beautifully wrapped wedding gift.

"Wait and unwrap it with Burt. I know you will love it. Shall I tell you what it is?"

"Yes, please."

Shirley had already guessed from the shape of the parcel, but she did not let on.

"It's the china teapot that you have always liked. Every time you've cleaned it I have watched the way you look at it and the spray of flowers on the side."

"Thank you so much. I'll always think of you whenever Burt and I use it," said the grateful young bride, her eyes sparkling with gratitude.

"You will be in good hands with that lovely young man," said Mrs. Brogan. "You and your....." she suddenly stopped talking, understanding that Shirley did not want anyone to know that she was pregnant, even though the 'shotgun wedding' gave it away.

"I would have loved to invite you and Mr. Brogan, but we just wanted a very small wedding."

"I know. I know. Now off you go, young lady. You don't want to keep your groom waiting at the church. You look simply lovely. Mr. Brogan has the car out front, on the street, ready to drive you. Here, let me pin this spray of flowers on your jacket. I gathered them this morning and then almost forgot to give them to you."

Mrs. Brogan pinned a small arrangement of several small flowers on to the shoulder of Shirley's suit.

"Why Shirley, the blue suit brings out the lovely blue of your eyes. You look like a film star."

Shirley giggled nervously at the compliment and hugged her employer, warmly. She impulsively kissed her on the cheek, all of her gratitude in that kiss for the many kindnesses during her stay as their live-in maid. With a quick check that she had her prayer book and handbag, together with a small bag for her over-night things, she walked out the front door for the last time and away from a home that she had come to love dearly.

Chapter Fifty

"When you realise you want to spend the rest of your life with somebody, you want the rest of your life to start as soon as possible." "When Harry Met Sally" (Movie)

He was waiting nervously for her at the church. As soon as he saw her, his face lit up and he offered his elbow to her, just like at the dance at the Embassy. She smiled shyly at him, as he escorted her to the church vestry. They could not be married in the Queen of Angels Catholic Church at Thebarton, as Burt was not a Catholic. But the vestry was allowed. The couple were disappointed, but the priest would not budge. Shirley looked around at the few supporters who were assembled for her wedding day. There was Jack and the adored Annie Mulvihill, Burt's aunt and uncle, Percy Gilfillan and Molly Brodie. They were not to be married for some years as Percy was still married to Phyllis. Also an old friend, Muriel Golding. It was 6:00 pm. There were no presents and no cards.

The bride looked at each person standing in the church vestry, allowing the memories they triggered to linger. Jack and Annie always treated her kindly and there was laughter wherever they went. Jack was the brother of her future mother-in-law and she marvelled at how different they were. She had visited their welcoming home three times with Burt and had loved the time spent with these relatives. They treated her as if she was someone special and made no fuss over the fact that she was so much younger than their nephew. She loved to sit in their deep, comfy chairs in their sitting room, sipping cups of tea like a lady, and munching on their delicious home-made biscuits. She remembered the highly polished lino floor and lovely carved buffet, displaying various treasures on top and hiding others inside. Everything looked lovingly cared for, including the couple who lived there.

Shirley felt a stab of pain as she thought of Burt's absent parents and how she would soon be living with them in the dark, unfriendly atmosphere they created. She quickly shook off the threatening thoughts and imagined herself tucked up in Burt's single bed, snuggling together with him and their love blocking out the meanness of his parents.

Her eyes fell on her father who had dressed up in his only suit, and given it a sponge and a press for the occasion. He seemed to be happy and sad all at once. She suspected that he was sorry that she and Burt could not move in with him, Molly and her mother, as Burt had requested. Even though Molly would have liked the extra money, there was no room. Shirley looked quickly past Molly. She wished her father would leave her and find someone more suitable. However, in spite of her youth, Shirley had quickly concluded he was a weak man who somehow was comfortable being controlled by two women. It seemed obvious to her now that Percy preferred someone else to make the hard decisions, pay the bills and take charge of his life for him.

At least she is here with my father, so that is something.

Shirley chose to look on the bright side, having learned this from her husband-to-be. She remembered how Percy's bride had lied on her marriage certificate, stating her age as six years younger, for Percy's benefit, and how she herself was about to lie on her marriage certificate as well.

Am I just like my mother? A wave of horror, then sadness swept over her. Horror at the thought of being anything like her poor mother and then sadness that her poor mother was locked in an institution and not present on her only child's wedding day. A huge lump in her throat threatened approaching tears and Shirley dug into her bag for the pretty lace handkerchief that her best friend, Rita, from St. Joseph's, had given her.

I miss you and I am thinking of you on my special day, she thought. *I wish you were here.* A tear finally found its way to her chin, and then another. She quickly blew her nose and wiped her face. Next, her eyes fell on Muriel, the elder sister of the Golding clan, who had all been at St. Joseph's with her. They had become her family, too. Memories came on wings, fluttering through her mind. Good friends, where relationships grew out of bad times. A sister that she never had, here to support her. One who knew her so well that she could sum up the true state of affairs and say nothing about it, knowing this would shame her. She had asked a few questions earlier, whispering a few words, but had sensed to back off from Shirley's tense response. She was a true big sister and she was strong. They had all looked up to her in the orphanage and she had never let them down. A strong sense of family warmed her as the young bride looked at Muriel.

The priest was talking. There was an awkward silence and Burt squeezed her hand. She answered, "I do." The ceremony was over quickly and they were married. They seemed to get away with the lie about her age, as no-one queried it, or asked for a birth certificate. The newly married couple thanked their friends for coming. Burt paid the priest and they made their way in a borrowed car to see Margaret and Walter. Burt wanted to do the right thing and take his bride to see his parents, even though they had chosen not to attend his wedding. He held her hand as they entered the house. The air was thick with tension and the young bride was aware that she had been verbally attacked during her last visit, just a few weeks ago. She trembled and he drew her closer.

"Well, here we are. The new Mr. and Mrs. Clough. What do you think Mum and Dad? Do we look the part?"

"Get that bung-eyed witch out of my house."

The old crone was on her feet pointing at Shirley, spitting out her never to be forgotten, venomous words.

"Now come on, Mum. You and I had a good talk and you agreed to be civil to my wife."

He spoke the last two words distinctly, giving his mother a clear message.

"Just get her out of my sight," spat out his jealous and bitter mother.

"We will be off in just a minute, but I want to pay you the ten bob that I owe you." He went to give the note to his father, but as quick as a greyhound, his mother stepped in between the two men and snatched the money.

"I'll have that, thank you." She spoke haughtily.

Shirley looked at Burt and saw him going through his wallet, frantically. He was visibly upset.

"We must go." He spoke urgently, and they were quickly out the door and in to the borrowed ute, speeding up the road. He explained to his new wife that he must have given the priest too much money as there was nothing left to pay for their wedding night at the Brighton Hotel. He drove back to the church where they had just been married and raced inside to find the priest, hoping and praying that he was still there and not out celebrating his windfall. When he saw the priest near the altar he pounced on him, startling the man of the cloth. Burt quickly explained his dilemma and the priest refunded the overpaid amount without hesitation.

He must have known that I overpaid him at the time, but chose not to say anything. Burt was hurt at the thought but willing to forgive him because he was so relieved to have his money returned. Normally, Burt had huge issues with the Catholic church. If the groom had not been refunded his money, the priest would have been in a spot of bother with this groom.

Someone to Watch Over Me

Happily this was not the case and Burt felt like hugging and kissing him with gratitude.

Relieved, he slid back into the seat next to Shirley, pecking her on the cheek, instead. Shirley saw his relief etched on his face and knew that this was all the money that he had in the world.

Chapter Fifty One

*"Vengeance to God alone belongs
But when I think of all my wrongs
My blood is liquid flame!"*

Sir Walter Scott. *Marmion*

He dragged himself back into the house after a long day up and down ladders, painting. His back was aching and his heart was heavy. It was not easy living with his parents at anytime, but it had been unbearable since his wife had moved in with them. Not that it was her fault. She had really tried to get on with his mother. It was all his mother's fault. Her jealousy was out of control. He braced himself for what might be ahead. As he opened the front door, he heard Shirley crying. He raced to her and took her into his arms. His mother was standing there, looking menacing with her hands on her hips, her feet astride in her slippers and looking fierce and threatening.

"I didn't know that she didn't want it cleaned," hiccuped the younger woman, hardly able to get the words out between sobs.

"What is this all about?" asked the exasperated young husband.

"She scrubbed my black pot. The one I always keep on the stove. She is stupid. A fool would know that you don't scrub a heavy black pot. It cooks better if you leave it black."

"I was only trying to help. All I know is cleaning and we always scrubbed the pots at the orphanage. I thought it would please you."

Someone to Watch Over Me

Shirley finally looked up at Burt, the tears still spilling down her face.

Then he saw. She had been battered in the face and was bruised and scratched. Ugly welts stood up under the scratches and the skin was broken in places. Her blind eye had been attacked and it was swollen and closed. It would look worse tomorrow. He made a dreadful sound, like a wounded animal as he grabbed Shirley and raced her out the back door, banging the screen door behind him, ferociously.

Anger rose up inside him like lava in a volcano. He had had enough. His mother must be dealt with. This could not go on. Shirley was vulnerable and she was pregnant with his baby. His body shook as he battled to contain his anger. He walked up and down around the vegetable patches to relieve his tension and then stumbled upon his beloved cricket cream pants and jumper, lying muddied and ruined in the dirt. Someone had pulled them, wet, from the clothesline and dragged them in the dust.

His mother of course, jealous of Shirley washing his clothes and claiming her territory back like a mad dog.

"Stay here darling, where you are safe. I won't be long."

Burt threw the door open and stood just inside the room. Light streamed in and he was silhouetted, looking like the avenging angel Gabriel. He stood with feet wide apart and arms crossed on his chest.

"You have wronged me deeply, mother. For years! You hurt someone I love, you hurt me! Never again, mother! Never again! One nasty word! One unkind action! Anything from you to hurt or harm my wife," and then he yelled for emphasis, "And you will never see me again. Never! You two will be thrown out of my house and on your own. Do you hear me?"

Margaret was speechless as she saw the fire in his eyes and the look of ferocious rage on his face. Her son had always been kind to her, no matter what was going on. He had never spoken to her like this before. She pulled herself together with indignation and was about to say, "How dare you" when she looked again at his face. She knew. He meant every word. If she did not change her ways, she would not see her beloved son again. She and Walter would have nowhere to live. He was her youngest child and her most adored. He had been so good to her and Walter. She didn't want to lose him. She hated Shirley so much for stealing her son's affection.

A heavy silence hung in the room like a London fog. They both stood like statues, glaring at each other. Finally Burt spoke again.

"I hope I have made myself clear!"

He walked out through the back door and found Shirley. She looked up into his face frantically, searching for reassurance and comfort. He cradled her in his arms and whispered words of love and protection, feeling her relax against him as she drew strength from him. He thought of her injuries again, and anger seethed inside his chest. He gently steered her back through the door into the kitchen.

"Mum and Dad, we are going out to visit Uncle Jack and Aunt Annie. I think my wife and I need some time with decent, caring people, for a change! I will ask if we can stay with them for a few days. Make sure my cricket creams are washed clean by the time we get back. If you are planning any nasty pay-backs, I suggest that you take stock and forget it. Living on the streets will be your reward for any further cruelty."

Neither his father or mother spoke a word.

He steered Shirley into their room to pack a few things, taking only a few minutes.

He stormed out of the house, banging the door behind him to punctuate his angry words, dragging Shirley with him as she held tightly to his hand. He had no idea of the time, but headed for the tram stop, hoping that one would come along quickly. One hand in his pocket, he jiggled the coins to see if he had the fare.

Someone to Watch Over Me

The two older people left behind were silent and motionless for some time. They both knew that things would never be the same again.

Someone to Watch Over Me

Chapter Fifty Two

"Grace comes into the SOUL, as the morning sun into the world; first a dawning; then a LIGHT; and at last in His full and excellent brightness." Thomas Adams.

"Yes, my love. I have found a little place for us. It is only small, but we can afford the rent. The landlady seems kind and she is alright with us having a baby on the way. She said that she may be able to baby-sit for us now and again. It's not perfect, Shirl, but it will be our own little place and you can fix it up however you like. The laundry is outside, and we share it, but I'm sure we can work around that. I can't wait to show it to you. It's at Henley Beach and not far from the beach, so we can get to take those sunset walks you dream about."

He was excited and she had never seen him quite so talkative. He had hardly drawn breath while sharing his thrilling news. She could sense the relief in him and understood that living with his parents had been as stressful for him as it had been for her. His mother had behaved herself since his threat to walk out of her life, but she had continued to make it clear that she did not like Shirley at all. The young teen-ager patted her tummy and thought of the three of them in their own home as a real family at last. That was all she needed in the world to make her happy. She felt rich. Rich in the things that mattered most to her. She knew without a doubt that her prayer for someone to watch over her had been answered beyond her wildest dreams in Burt, her champion.

There was much to do before the birth, and she could busy herself preparing the place for her little one. Burt had managed to get some left over paint and the landlady had agreed to his painting out the place before they moved in. He planned to do it over the next week-end, and they would move in a couple of days after that. Burt placed his hand over hers, on her stomach, indicating that he knew where her thoughts had been.

"What about a cricket team sweetheart? I always wanted lots of kids. What do you think about that?"

Shirley smiled with joy, and then allowed a nervous frown to crease her forehead. She was thinking this time of all the screaming, needy children in the orphanage.

"One at a time Burt. Let's see how we go with this one first."

They chuckled together as they looked to their future with hope and love, determining to walk into the sunrise, letting the light shine brighter and brighter as the sun rose in their lives as they walked away from the shadows of the past.

Epilogue

Shirley and Burt produced six babies in six years and they needed to move several times to accommodate their expanding family. Burt worked extremely hard as a master plumber, establishing his own business. He proudly displayed in his front garden, a sign with the words "B.J. CLOUGH - MASTER PLUMBER." He did not enjoy the work, but endured the challenges as it fed his rapidly growing family.

He purchased a blue Holden utility for the business and this needed to double as the family car. This meant that wherever they went, in all weather, the children travelled in the back of the ute, under a tarpaulin when it was cold or it rained. Sadly, their third daughter, when only four, fell out of the utility along Port Road, sustaining head injuries and being treated at the Adelaide Children's Hospital. Thankfully she recovered, but the accident was a dreadful trauma for her and left scars on her forehead and caused for her a life-long struggle with anxiety. It was also a dreadful trauma for her father, who felt responsible, but did not have the means to purchase two cars.

Shirley was twenty three when they had their sixth child. Her body did not have time to fully recover between each baby and she was tired and overwhelmed. She found it very hard looking after so many children, all needing attention, and their ages being so close. One would become ill and they all became ill. She could not cope and would lose control. Burt was working in the country a great deal of the time, desperately accepting whatever work he could obtain. He worked often with his father and brother painting, when they managed to get work, even though it was usually a long way from home.

Burt hated being away from his family but had no choice. He needed to bring in money to feed and clothe his wife and children. He worked long and exhausting hours, often in very trying conditions, going without himself so that his family would be provided for. He wrote many letters to Shirley, expressing his love and encouraging her with promises to be home soon. He begged for letters back, but Shirley's literacy skills were poor and so he didn't receive many.

Twelve years after their son was born, which was a great joy to them after five girls, Shirley gave birth to another daughter. They were thrilled to be blessed in this way and celebrated having seven children. Shirley now had a large family - making up for the longing in her heart as a little girl.

By now Burt had established another business, giving up the plumbing that he hated and working as a tiler, using his creative talent. His business was called Northern Tiling Company and he was kept very busy as the work flooded in. He hired a couple of young men and they enjoyed each other's company, with lots of joking and great camaraderie. No matter how difficult things would get, Burt always found something to laugh about.

He continued to support his parents throughout their lives, setting them up in a house in Kilburn, and always treating them with love and respect. He refused to speak a word against them.

Shirley was very proud of her large family and the different skills her children demonstrated. Some inherited her musical ability, two inherited Burt's artistic flair and became artists, some worked in offices, two as teachers, one as a nurse, one in sales in her own business and their son as a builder. Their mother's freedom came in small steps and her self-confidence grew as she ventured more and more from the house. She now had her own income as she cleaned houses, putting into practice the skills she had learned as a maid. Exchanging her bike for a small car was a huge thrill. Cake decorating was a hobby that she embraced and in which she excelled. She loved it and her self confidence grew. Next came millinery, in a time when hats were very much in fashion. She had a wonderful time going to class and creating works of art. Her next challenge was lawn bowls and Shirley found that she had a natural talent, winning many trophies and loving the social side of the sport as well. When she and Burt travelled with their caravan, they loved to play bowls in different country towns, making friends as they went. Church attendance became part of their family life in 1957 and this impacted the large and busy family positively. Suddenly there were social things to attend. Church services, Bible studies, choir practices, youth groups, sing-alongs after church, Christian Endeavour, picnics and sports.

Life became full and the atmosphere of the home became more harmonious. Shirley took a while to feel safe around 'religion.' She resisted being involved as the nuns had told her how wicked the protestants were and that she would be smitten should she even enter one of their churches. She soon realised that this did not happen and the family laughed together at the happy outcome after her first church service in a non-Catholic church.

One traumatic outcome for Shirley from her tragic childhood was the fracturing of her personality and the development of multiple personality disorder. Her family was told that this was a result of severe trauma, like imprisonment, child sexual abuse, physical abuse, deprivation and neglect, all of which Shirley experienced as a child. The development of other personalities helped her to survive the abuse as she told herself it was not happening to her, but to some other poor girl. Towards the end of her life she became the authentic Shirley, receiving healing from the past. She found the strength, with God's help, to forgive the nuns, the Catholic Church, the old man in Carrieton, her parents and in her own words, "I had to forgive God too for letting those horrible things happen to me." Shirley was set free.

Shirley and Burton James were married for fifty five years and were not separated, in spite of a sometimes volatile relationship, until Burt passed away in 1997. Shirley had nursed her beloved Burt for the last few years of his life, after Alzheimers changed him. Her doctor tried in vain to persuade her to leave him in the nursing home, but always independent and feisty, she had Burt discharged and brought him home. It was not easy for them. When it was beyond her, Burt saw his last days back in a nursing home, not far from their home and Shirley insisted on doing all of his washing and visited him daily, tending to him, feeding him, reading to him and holding his hand.

Their love story had times of sunshine and times of shadow, but the last chapter painted a true portrait of their deep and enduring love for each other.

Her years on her own as a widow were lonely and difficult and many tears were shed over the loss of her Burtie. No matter how many times her family visited, nothing ever filled her empty cup for her beloved husband.

Shirley was blessed with many grand-children and great grand-children. Those prayers to the subject of that grubby photograph of Jesus kept under her pillow for years were well and truly answered. She had the family that she craved. Nothing else mattered. Material things held no real value for her. It was always family where her treasure lay. The only jewellery she owned that was real and not 'costume' were her rings. It was impossible to convince her to spend any money on herself. She always had a problem with self esteem but her God esteemed her and blessed her with the things that really mattered. When she was fearful of dying and not being accepted by her Heavenly Father and convinced that she was not good enough for heaven, He sent just the right person to pray with her and reassure her from the Bible the truth that none of us are good enough and that is why we need a Saviour, Jesus.

Not long before Shirley went to heaven, she was blessed with an incredible experience. She couldn't wait to tell someone and had to wait for a visitor for this to happen. That visitor was her eldest daughter. Paralysed down one side for the last year of her life, Shirley was excited and animated by what had happened. Lying in her bed, she raised herself up on one arm, leaning in and bursting with joy like a child at Christmas. Her daughter quickly pulled up a chair and leaned in to her, taking her hand and listening to her story.

"Two huge angels came into my room"

"Wow. Did they? What were they like?"

"They were massive. Very tall. They were lovely."

"Did you see wings?"

"No wings. They were both dressed in white."

"How wonderful! What did they say?"

"They told me that they would be coming back soon to carry me to heaven. They said not to be afraid, it is going to be wonderful in heaven. Then they left."

Her daughter was speechless.

"Jesus came into my room too."

"At the same time as the angels?"

"No. A different time. He is so beautiful."

"Wow Mum. I don't know what to say. What did He say to you?"

"He was so kind to me. He came up close to my bed. He's absolutely lovely."

She was beaming with joy and full of love and peace.

"He told me not to be scared but that heaven is a beautiful place and I will love it there. He told me all about it. He said He loves me and I am truly His. He said that He would be coming back with the angels and would escort me to heaven Himself. He said that to me. I am going to heaven very soon. I can't wait. I'm so excited. I want to go right now!"

Excited she was. So excited and so reassured that there is not the slightest doubt in her daughter's mind that this was a real experience and something gracious and reassuring that she had been blessed with. It has touched her daughter deeply to experience such an amazing episode in her mother's life. Shirley now knew where she was going and kept crying out to her Heavenly Father and to Jesus in prayer whenever the pain and discomfort overwhelmed her during the last week of her life.

Shirley, with no middle name, rejected and mistreated and misunderstood and broken was accepted and loved and watched over by her amazing Jesus who brought Burt into her life, blessed her with seven children whom she loved passionately and then many grand and great-grandchildren. She had her longed for family and also belonged to the family of God forever in heaven. A truly blessed woman. Someone who was watched over and loved and will be for eternity. Set free from pain and a body that was worn out and now with her beloved Burt forever.

Carried in the arms of huge angels and escorted by the King of Kings and Lord of Lords to her new home, as a precious and valued member of the family of God.

Class Action

Shirley was awarded $20,000 in 2008 for the ill-treatment received whilst in care in St. Joseph's Orphanage at Largs Bay.

Sadly, she refused to spend any of this money on herself, no matter how encouraged she was to do so. Her clothes were all second-hand and she would rather go without herself, in order for her children to benefit.

State Government Inquiry Into Children In State Care (Mullighan Inquiry)

In 2004 the Parliament of South Australia enacted legislation to establish a Commission of Inquiry into Children in State Care.

Commissioner Ted Mullighan QC presented the reports of the Children in State Care. He interviewed a huge number of such children. Shirley Clough was one of them. He showed her empathy, respect and compassion. He told her that she was the oldest at eighty one to come forward. He praised her generously and told her daughter that she could be proud of her mother, as she had survived and had successfully raised a family. He explained that this was not an easy accomplishment for someone who had suffered the traumatic experiences of her childhood.

Her interview with the Hon. Ted Mullighan QC was an uplifting experience for Shirley. The respect that he showed her and the kindness he demonstrated was a huge encouragement to her.

The fact that he had a high position, and yet treated her with warmth and understanding brought great comfort to her. Over and over again she mentioned how nice Mr. Mullighan had been to her.

He made a great impact on her, and on her self-esteem.

Her obvious appreciation at being on the receiving end of affirmation from a man who had been a Supreme Court Judge and was now a Commissioner, heading up the State Inquiry, enabled her to gain a sense of worth that had until then escaped her.

Someone to Watch Over Me

IRENE GLEESON FOUNDATION

Any proceeds from the sale of this book will be directed to the Irene Gleeson Foundation, which was a favourite of Shirley's.

The Amazing IGF Story

In 1991, Irene Gleeson (RIP), an Australian grandmother, heard about children being abducted by Joseph Kony's Lord's Resistance Army (LRA) in Northern Uganda. Irene was concerned about the plight of the children and felt God's call on her life to rescue them.

She sold everything she owned including her beachside home in Sydney, towed her modest caravan to Uganda, and used the proceeds of the sale to begin a Full Daycare school in Kitgum, Uganda. A school teacher by trade, Irene began by teaching fifty children to write their names in the dust under a mango tree. Irene lived through fifteen years of war, attacks, poverty and refugee camp life, and spent a third of her life with the people of northern Uganda.

Her first school under a tree has grown into four Primary and two Technical and Business schools that feed, medicate and educate over 4,000 children and youth daily. A health program has evolved to keep children and parents healthy, including a maternity hospital currently under construction, and village and community health initiatives. A 1,500 member Community Church has grown at the main campus and offers spiritual healing restoration and support to members of the local community with a vibrant youth, women, children, hospital, prison and discipleship ministry.

In addition, IGF manages 91.5 Mighty Fire FM, a community radio station that broadcasts educational programs and local gospel music. With over a million listeners, Mighty Fire is the second biggest and most influential radio station in northern Uganda.

Irene was declared a national hero by the President and Parliament of Uganda. She has also been honoured by the Australian government. In 2009 she received the Honour of Officer of the Order of Australia for "service to international relations particularly through sustained aid for children affected by war and HIV/AIDS in northern Uganda" and media outlets began to dub her Australia's Mother Teresa.

Irene passed away on 21st July 2013 after a courageous battle with cancer. What a great legacy she left for us to continue. **Irene Gleeson Foundation employs 300 Ugandan staff, led by Executive Director John Paul Kaffasi, who are faithfully continuing Irene's dream of bringing lasting change to the people of north Uganda.**

Visit the website for further information and to sponsor a child at *irenegleesonfoundation.com*

From the Author.....

We are all redeemable!

My broken and damaged mother's story of healing was a perfect example of the miracles that God can work in someone's heart.

As Shirley recognised her need to accept all that Jesus Christ accomplished for her on the cross, so can you. As she journeyed through forgiving those who had abused and shamefully mistreated her, so can you. With God's help. Her reward was the freedom she experienced and the relationship with her Heavenly Father that she embraced.

May you be encouraged by Shirley's story that Jesus can take any life and redeem, heal and restore. Your brokenness is not too hard for Him to deal with. He works miracles, just as He did with my dear mother.

Following are some Bible verses. The first one my mother quoted often:

We love Him because He first loved us. 1 John 4:19 NKJV

God did not send His Son into the world to condemn the world, but to save the world through Him. John 3 : 17 NIV

If anyone is in Christ he is a new creation, the old has gone, the new has come.   11 Corinthians 5 : 17 NIV

You will show me the way of life, granting me the joy of your presence and the pleasures of living with you forever. Psalm16:11 NIV

Satisfy us in the morning with your unfailing love, that we may sing for joy and be glad all our days. Psalm 90:14 NIV

Jesus said, "I am the resurrection and the life. Whoever believes in me will live, even though they die." John 11:25 NIV

www.ingramcontent.com/pod-product-compliance
Lightning Source LLC
Chambersburg PA
CBHW071902290426
44110CB00013B/1253